Lifestyle Medicine

Dedication

This book is dedicated to all Lifestyle Medicine Physicians, Professionals, Practitioners, Group Consultation Facilitators, Researchers, Students, and all the patients they serve.

We give thanks for the enabling grace to complete this work.

Ifeoma Monye, Adaeze Ifezulike, Karen Adamson, and Fraser Birrell.

Lifestyle Medicine

Essential MCQs for Certification in Lifestyle Medicine

IFEOMA MONYE

Regional Director, BSLM and Board-Certified Lifestyle Medicine Physician
Sessional GP, Berkshire Healthcare NHS Foundation Trust
United Kingdom
Chief Consultant Family Physician, National Hospital Abuja, Nigeria
Brookfield Centre for Lifestyle Medicine, Abuja, Nigeria
Founding President, Society of Lifestyle Medicine of Nigeria

ADAEZE IFEZULIKE

Regional Director, BSLM and Board-Certified Lifestyle Medicine Physician, GP NHS Grampian Aberdeen
United Kingdom

KAREN ADAMSON

Regional Director of BSLM Lifestyle Medicine Physician
Consultant Physician, Diabetologist and Endocrinologist
Clinical Director of Medicine and Associated Services
NHS Lothian, United Kingdom

FRASER BIRRELL

Director of Science & Research, BSLM, Editor-in Chief of Lifestyle Medicine, Engagement Lead Centre for Integrated Research into Musculoskeletal Ageing
Newcastle University, Consultant & Senior Lecturer
Northumbria Healthcare NHS Foundation Trust
United Kingdom

WILEY Blackwell

This edition first published 2022
© 2022 John Wiley & Sons Ltd

The right of Ifeoma Monye, Adaeze Ifezulike, Karen Adamson, and Fraser Birrell to be identified as the authors of this work has been asserted in accordance with law.

Registered Office(s)
John Wiley & Sons, Inc., 111 River Street, Hoboken, NJ 07030, USA
John Wiley & Sons Ltd, The Atrium, Southern Gate, Chichester, West Sussex, PO19 8SQ, UK

Editorial Office
9600 Garsington Road, Oxford, OX4 2DQ, UK

For details of our global editorial offices, customer services, and more information about Wiley products visit us at www.wiley.com.

Wiley also publishes its books in a variety of electronic formats and by print-on-demand. Some content that appears in standard print versions of this book may not be available in other formats.

Library of Congress Cataloging-in-Publication Data
Names: Monye, Ifeoma, author. | Ifezulike, Adaeze, author. | Adamson, Karen, author. | Birrell, Fraser, author.
Title: Lifestyle medicine : essential MCQs for certification in lifestyle medicine / Ifeoma Monye, Adaeze Ifezulike, Karen Adamson, Fraser Birrell.
Description: First edition. | Hoboken, NJ : Wiley-Blackwell, 2022. | Includes index.
Identifiers: LCCN 2021027293 (print) | LCCN 2021027294 (ebook) | ISBN 9781119795919 (paperback) | ISBN 9781119795926 (adobe pdf) | ISBN 9781119795964 (epub)
Subjects: MESH: Preventive Medicine–methods | Life Style | Healthy Lifestyle | Risk Reduction Behavior | Health Promotion–methods
Classification: LCC RA427.8 (print) | LCC RA427.8 (ebook) | NLM WA 108| DDC 362.1–dc23
LC record available at https://lccn.loc.gov/2021027293
LC ebook record available at https://lccn.loc.gov/2021027294

Cover Design: Wiley
Cover Images: © Instants/Getty Images, © Deagreez/Getty Images, © digitalskillet/Getty Images, © OksanaKiian/Getty Images, © Ridofranz/Getty Images, © PeopleImages/Getty Images
Author Photos: Courtesy of the Authors

Set in 10/12pt STIX Two Text by Straive, Pondicherry, India

10 9 8 7 6 5 4 3 2 1

Contents

Each chapter of questions is followed by answers and a brief note about the answer to each question. This is supported by selected references and tip boxes, again provided by the chapter to support learning.

Acknowledgments

When Dr Ifeoma Monye and Dr Adaeze Ifezulike were preparing for the first-ever Board Certification examination in Lifestyle Medicine, in the United Kingdom, they faced a daunting task of finding suitable revision materials. As pioneers for that examination in August 2018, all candidates had the same challenge! Where to find a multiple-choice revision book to test your knowledge of Lifestyle Medicine and aid revision?

Therefore, at the end of the examination, they decided to create a resource that future candidates for this examination and indeed other Lifestyle Medicine examinations will use to make revision easier. In the course of securing a publisher and putting together the best possible book, they invited Dr Karen Adamson, Founding Director of the British Society of Lifestyle Medicine and Dr Fraser Birrell, Founding Editor-in-Chief of the Wiley open access journal *Lifestyle Medicine* to co-author.

We all want to thank the Chairman of the British Society of Lifestyle Medicine and now President of the World Lifestyle Medicine Council, Dr Rob Lawson for reviewing the book, providing feedback, and his support of the MCQ Book.

We are all also grateful to Dr Lilach Maleskey, President of the Israeli Association of Lifestyle Medicine for reviewing the book and making very useful suggestions which has helped enrich the final product.

We appreciate the support from Stephan Herzog, the Executive Director of the International Board of Lifestyle Medicine and the useful suggestions he provided.

Finally, we are all indebted to our families who had to put up with the disruption caused by the long hours, days, weeks, months of preparation, while we researched, wrote, edited, and proofed this book. Without your support, patience and understanding, we may not have made it this far.

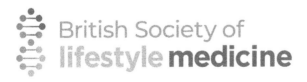

Foreword

Lifestyle as Medicine has never been so important, in the presence of the syndemic era of both infectious and chronic diseases. With the relatively recent arrival of a myriad of chronic diseases and the seeming difficulty of established health care to deal with them effectively, it is entirely appropriate to use Lifestyle Medicine to manage, reverse, and prevent the steady march of modern diseases around the world. Addressing the upstream causes, or metabolic inflammatory determinants of these diseases, is clearly the way ahead and is rooted in the accepted wisdom of evidence-based science. These upstream determinants include social, environmental, economic, and more readily understood areas such as inactivity, poor nutrition, lack of emotional wellbeing, sleep disturbance, and exposure to toxic substances.

This very timely book will test you in some of these areas – and hopefully will encourage you to learn more about topics in which you feel less confident. And, in time, steer you towards seeking a solid qualified grounding in this effective and satisfying approach to health care. A meaningful biopsychosocial engagement with your patient or client will bear huge dividends not only for your patient or client, but also for the wider systems of health care in which you work.

So, enjoy working your way through this book of MCQs, learn lots from further reading of referenced material, and celebrate by introducing changes into your clinical or professional practice. A positive experience not to be missed!

Dr Rob Lawson FRCGP Dip IBLM/BSLM

Chairman, British Society of Lifestyle Medicine

President, European Lifestyle Medicine Council

Chairman, World Lifestyle Medicine Council

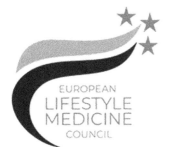

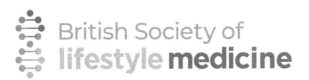

CHAPTER 1

Introduction to Lifestyle Medicine

Introduction

Lifestyle Medicine is a new and evolving speciality in Medicine. It is a distinct speciality aimed at treating the root cause of most chronic diseases using the strongest evidence-based modalities available. Current approaches to medicine and health care offer inadequate solutions to the problems we face. Lifestyle Medicine seeks to address these issues to improve the health and wellbeing of individuals and societies. This chapter covers the definition of Lifestyle Medicine and provides some questions to test candidates understanding of the difference between Lifestyle Medicine and other disciplines such as Conventional, Complementary, and Alternative medicine (CAM), and Integrative and Functional Medicine, to mention but a few.

1. Lifestyle Medicine is best defined by which of the following?
   a. A branch of alternative medicine
   b. A new field of medicine where lifestyle interventions are effective in the prevention, treatment and, rarely, reversal of diseases
   c. Evidence-based use of whole food, plant-based dietary lifestyle, regular physical activity, restorative sleep, stress management, avoidance of toxic substances such as tobacco and alcohol and supportive social connections for a healthy life
   d. The application of medical, behavioural, motivational, and environmental principles in the management of lifestyle-related health problems in a non-clinical setting

Lifestyle Medicine: Essential MCQs for Certification in Lifestyle Medicine, First Edition.
Ifeoma Monye, Adaeze Ifezulike, Karen Adamson and Fraser Birrell.
© 2022 John Wailey & Sons Ltd. Published 2022 by John Wiley & Sons Ltd.

2. Lifestyle Medicine is most appropriately described in which of the following ways?
   a. The integration of lifestyle practices into conventional medicine to lower the risk for chronic disease
   b. The integration of lifestyle practices into conventional medicine to eliminate conventional medical practice
   c. The integration of lifestyle practices in the form of complementary therapy
   d. The integration of lifestyle practices in the form of alternative therapy

3. Which of the following best describes the practice of Lifestyle Medicine?
   a. A practice that does not include medications
   b. A practice that involves environmental and dietary interventions
   c. A practice where medications, rather than behaviour change, form a significant part of the management
   d. A practice where self-management is not an essential component

4. Which of the following is a major component of Lifestyle Medicine?
   a. Cessation of all medications
   b. Ozone therapy
   c. Physical activity
   d. Use of supplements

5. Which of the following best describes a key component of the practice of Lifestyle Medicine?
   a. Emphasis on diagnostic laboratory tests
   b. Emphasis on vitamin supplements
   c. Pharmaceuticals as first line of treatment
   d. Use of whole food plant-based nutrition

6. Which of the following best describes the place of coaching in Lifestyle Medicine?
   a. It is not an essential component in Lifestyle Medicine
   b. It has not been found to be effective in depression management
   c. It can be used to improve personal lifestyle choices regarding weight management and physical activity or sleep
   d. The coach prescribes the best management for the patient

7. Which of the following most closely describes the best practice in Lifestyle Medicine?
   a. Emotional wellness plays a minimal role
   b. Nutrition must follow a named diet to yield lasting results
   c. Medication remains the mainstay of management
   d. Sleep prescription is an important pillar in the management of many chronic diseases

8. Which of the following is most distinctive of Lifestyle Medicine practice?
   a. It places emphasis on behavioural change
   b. It places emphasis on non-behavioural interventions
   c. It requires a multi-professional team
   d. The doctor is the only important clinician in the team

9. Which of the following most appropriately describes a Lifestyle Medicine setting?
   a. Inpatient surgical care centre
   b. Primary, secondary, or tertiary care clinics that incorporate group consultations in the management of their patients
   c. Super-specialist diagnostic centre
   d. Tertiary consultant-delivered service

10. Which of the following best describes primary care-shared medical appointments (a form of group consultation) in Lifestyle Medicine?
    a. Patients often complain of confidentiality issues
    b. Research has shown that patients do not like this approach compared to conventional single-person appointment
    c. Shared medical appointments offer time and space to empower patients to self-manage
    d. These are not an ideal approach for behavioural change

11. The most compelling evidence for the effectiveness of therapeutic lifestyle change comes from which of the following?
    a. Studies of annual therapeutic lifestyle change clinic visit programs
    b. Studies of intensive therapeutic lifestyle change programs
    c. Studies of monthly therapeutic lifestyle change clinic visit programs
    d. Studies of non-intensive therapeutic lifestyle change programs

12. Which of these most appropriately explains the difference between Lifestyle Medicine and other types of practice?
    a. It is distinctly different from all the other categories of medicine
    b. It is the same as Alternative Medicine
    c. It is the same as Complementary Medicine
    d. It is the same as Functional Medicine

13. In understanding Lifestyle Medicine and Integrative Medicine, which of the following best explains their relationship?
    a. Both are patient-centred and involve personalized care
    b. Both place the same emphasis on behavioural change

    c. They are exactly the same

    d. They do not have any common components

14. In understanding Lifestyle Medicine and Functional Medicine, which of these is the most appropriate statement?

    a. Both place emphasis on vitamin supplements

    b. Both are forms of Alternative Medicine

    c. Functional Medicine is concerned with interactions between the environment, gastrointestinal, endocrine, and immune systems to create individualized care

    d. They do not have anything in common

15. Concerning Lifestyle Medicine and Conventional Medicine, which of these statements best describes the differences?

    a. Both place the same emphasis on behavioural intervention

    b. Conventional Medicine places emphasis on restoring function by addressing the root cause through individualized treatment

    c. Lifestyle Medicine, unlike Conventional Medicine, emphasizes cellular metabolism and control of oxidative stress

    d. Unlike Lifestyle Medicine, in Conventional Medicine, apart from complying with the prescribed medications or surgery, patients are not required to make significant changes

16. In the therapeutic approaches used in Lifestyle Medicine, which of these therapeutic interventions has been most appropriately represented?

    a. Cognitive Behavioural Therapy is seldom used

    b. Group consultations have been found to be effective

    c. Lifestyle Medicine approaches have not been found to be effective in the management of communicable diseases

    d. Motivational counselling is more effective than medications in severe depression

17. Comparing Lifestyle Medicine and Preventive Medicine, which of these best compares their approaches?

    a. Lifestyle Medicine practice is the same as Preventive Medicine in approach

    b. Medication is the 'end' in both fields of Medicine

    c. Personalized care is a key feature in both the fields of Medicine

    d. Preventive Medicine, unlike Lifestyle Medicine, emphasizes population-based interventions

18. Which of the following is a key process in health coaching for behavioural change in Lifestyle Medicine?

    a. Assessing the client's readiness for change

    b. Changing the lifestyle of the client

c. Enforcing behavioural change in the client

d. Setting goals for the client

19. Which of the following is the most appropriate behaviour change technique for the behaviour change process?

a. In all stages, use motivational interviewing

b. In all stages, use positive psychology

c. In the early stages, use cognitive behavioural therapy

d. In the later stages, use motivational interviewing

20. Which of the following best reflects physician competencies for prescribing Lifestyle Medicine?

a. Ideally, physicians will role-model and practice healthy personal behaviours

b. Physician helps patients sustain healthy lifestyle practices with no need to refer to other specialities

c. Physician's engagement with patients has not been shown to improve patient outcome

d. The healthcare provider should avoid engagement with the patient

21. In Physician Competencies in Lifestyle Medicine, which of the following best explains the important processes involved in the assessment of a patient?

a. Assessment of the employer's readiness and willingness is more important than family readiness and willingness

b. Assessment of environmental factors is the most important aspect

c. Assessment of family readiness and willingness is more important than the client's readiness and willingness

d. Assessment of social, psychological, and biological predispositions and the desired health outcome is very important

22. Health coaching in Lifestyle Medicine is more likely to succeed in which of the following situations?

a. Readiness of the patients and their community to make a health behaviour change

b. Readiness of the patients and their employer to make health behaviour change

c. Readiness of the patients and their family to make health behaviour change

d. Readiness of the patients and members of their support group to make a health behaviour change

23. Which of the following best describes the intensity component of the Lifestyle Medicine treatment intensity program?

a. Amount of contact hours during the program

b. Amount of days spent on the program

    c. Amount of physical activities on the program

    d. Amount of whole food plant-based options in the program

24. A 58-year-old man, diagnosed with Type 2 Diabetes 20 years ago, recently moves into the area and registers as a new patient in the primary care clinic. His BMI is 40. He has dyslipidaemia, severe left hip pain, and is desperate to have Lifestyle Medicine interventions for his condition. For the past five years, his treatment consists of Soluble Insulin, Metformin, and Atorvastatin. Based on the current evidence, which of the following will be the most effective option of therapeutic lifestyle intervention treatment for him now?

    a. Intensive therapeutic lifestyle change treatment

    b. Intensive therapeutic lifestyle change treatment followed by therapeutic lifestyle change

    c. Non-intensive therapeutic lifestyle change treatment

    d. Non-intensive therapeutic lifestyle change treatment followed by therapeutic lifestyle change

25. In the scientific foundation of the Healthy Doctor = Healthy Patient project (Frank et al. 2013), which of the following most accurately represents the findings in this study?

    a. Counselling patients makes a difference in patients' habits and in their health

    b. North American physicians tend to live just as long as their peers

    c. Physicians live longer than their contemporaries because they have access to better medical care

    d. Physicians with poor health habits are more likely to advise their patients about preventive habits

Answers

1. C The website of the American College of Lifestyle Medicine provides a definition that states that 'Lifestyle Medicine involves the use of evidence-based lifestyle therapeutic approaches such as a predominantly whole food, plant-based diet, regular physical activity, adequate sleep, stress management, avoidance of risky substance use, and other non-drug modalities, to prevent, treat, and oftentimes reverse the lifestyle-related chronic disease that is all too prevalent'. In the 2017 edition of Egger's textbook, Lifestyle Medicine: Lifestyle, the Environment, and Preventive Medicine in Health and Disease, he defines Lifestyle Medicine as 'The application of environmental, behavioural (sic), medical, and motivational principles to the management of lifestyle-related health problems in a clinical and/or public health setting (Rippe 2019, pp. 961–962)'.

2. A Rippe defines Lifestyle Medicine as 'The integration of lifestyle practices into conventional medicine to lower the risk for chronic disease and, if the disease is already present, to serve as an adjunct to therapy' (Rippe 2019, pp. 961–962).

3. B There have been several definitions of Lifestyle Medicine by various schools of thought across the global community. The preferred definition may be that authored by Sanger, Katz, Dysinger, and others published in late 2014 in the International Journal of Clinical Practice: 'Lifestyle Medicine is the evidence-based practice of helping individuals and communities with comprehensive lifestyle changes (including nutrition, physical activity, stress management, social support, and environmental exposures) to help prevent, treat, and even reverse the progression of chronic diseases by addressing the underlying cause'.

4. C The overall benefits of physical activity on health include higher health-related fitness, higher control and maintenance of a healthy weight, less risk of disabling medical conditions and less chronic disease rates than people who are inactive. Physical inactivity is the fourth leading risk factor for global mortality. It is the cause of 1 in 10 premature deaths. Ozone therapy is not a component of Lifestyle Medicine. There is no emphasis on the use of supplements in Lifestyle Medicine. Evidence-based medication use is sometimes used as adjunct to Lifestyle Medicine treatment (Kelly and Shull 2019, pp. 187–191).

5. D A key component of the practice of Lifestyle Medicine is the use of whole food plant-based nutrition. Several studies have proved that plant-based nutrition prevents, treats, and oftentimes reverses the course of certain diseases such as hyperlipidaemia, hypertension, coronary artery disease (Ornish et al. 1990), Type 2 Diabetes Mellitus (Barnard et al. 2009), certain cancers (Kelly and Shull 2019, p. 125). A recent EAT-Lancet Commission series on healthy diets from sustainable food systems, 'Food in the Anthropocene' has also highlighted the benefits to the planet of a mainly plant-based diet (Willett et al. 2019; Tips Box 1.1), which inextricably links health and sustainable development.

TIPS BOX 1.1 | Key Messages from 'Food in the Anthropocene'

1. Unhealthy and unsustainably produced food poses a global risk to people and the planet. > 820 million people have insufficient food and many more consume an unhealthy diet that contributes to premature death and morbidity. Global food production is the largest pressure caused by humans on Earth, threatening local ecosystems and the stability of the Earth system.

2. Current dietary trends, combined with projected population growth to about 10 billion by 2050, will exacerbate risks to people and planet.

3. Transformation to healthy diets from sustainable food systems is necessary to achieve both UN Sustainable Development Goals and the Paris Agreement. Scientific targets for healthy diets/sustainable food production are needed to guide a Great Food Transformation.

4. Healthy diets have an appropriate caloric intake and consist of a diversity of plant-based foods, low amounts of animal source foods, unsaturated > saturated fats, and small amounts (if any) of refined grains, highly processed foods/added sugars.

5. Transformation to healthy diets by 2050 will require substantial dietary shifts, including a greater than 50% reduction in global consumption of unhealthy foods such as red meat and sugar, and a greater than 100% increase in consumption of healthy foods such as nuts, fruits, vegetables, and legumes.

6. Dietary changes from current diets to healthy diets are likely to substantially benefit human health, averting ~10.8–11.6 million deaths/year: a reduction of 19.0–23.6%

7. Sustainable food production needs to operate within the food systems' safe operating space at all scales on Earth. So, production for ~10 billion people should use no additional land, safeguard existing biodiversity, reduce consumptive water use/manage water responsibly, substantially reduce nitrogen/phosphorus pollution, produce zero CO_2 emissions, and no methane/nitrous oxide emission increase.

8. Transformation to sustainable food production by 2050 will require ≥ 75% reduction of yield gaps, global redistribution of nitrogen/phosphorus fertilizer use, phosphorus recycling, radical improvements in efficiency of fertilizer/water use, rapid implementation of agricultural mitigation options to reduce greenhouse-gas emissions, land management practices shifting agriculture from a carbon source to a sink, and a fundamental shift in production priorities.

9. The scientific targets for healthy diets from sustainable food systems are intertwined with all UN Sustainable Development Goals. For example, achieving these targets will depend on providing high-quality primary health care that integrates family planning and education on healthy diets. These targets and the Sustainable Development Goals on freshwater, climate, land, oceans, and biodiversity will be achieved through strong commitment to global partnerships and actions.

10. Achieving healthy diets from sustainable food systems for everyone will require substantial shifts towards healthy dietary patterns, large reductions in food losses and waste, and major improvements in food production practices.

Source: Willett et al. (2019).

6. C Health coaching in Lifestyle Medicine assesses the readiness for change, collaboratively establishing client goals, evaluating successful steps and self-limiting patterns, reassessing and modifying goals, articulating insights gained, and formulating post-coaching plan to sustain changes that promote health and wellness. Research has shown that patients who received coaching services demonstrated significant improvements in both physical as well as mental health, with reduction in chronic disease markers (HbA1c, blood pressure, and LDL cholesterol) that persisted one year after completion of the health coaching intervention.

Health coaching is an essential component of the practice of Lifestyle Medicine. It has been found to be effective in the treatment of mild-moderate depression. The coach does not prescribe a management plan for the client. Health coaching can be used to improve personal lifestyle choices regarding weight management and physical activity or sleep (Rippe 2019, p. 236).

7. D The main pillars of Lifestyle Medicine include Nutrition, Physical Activity, Sleep, Stress Management, Avoidance of Tobacco, Alcohol, and other harmful substances' Use, Social Connectedness, and Positive Psychology. Behavioural change is the mainstay of management. Nutrition needs to be plant-based and does not need to follow any particular named diet such as Mediterranean, Atkins, Paleo's, etc. Emotional wellness is a key component in the practice of Lifestyle Medicine (Rippe 2019, p. 964).

8. A Lifestyle Medicine places emphasis on behavioural change. This is the most distinctive aspect of the principles and practice of Lifestyle Medicine.

Behaviour change is the foundational activity through which Lifestyle Medicine works. Lifestyle Medicine often needs a multi-professional team, but behavioural change is the distinction from other specialities. All team members are equally important in the management of the patient (Rippe 2019, p. 193).

9. B A typical setting for a Lifestyle Medicine Clinic could be in a Primary, Secondary, or Tertiary clinic that incorporates the typical one-to-one consultation and group consultations in the management of patients. The practice of Lifestyle Medicine does not require a super-specialist diagnostic centre, nor is it typically a tertiary consultant-delivered service. Lifestyle Medicine involves significant evidence-based changes in behaviours that affect health by a multidisciplinary team whose members have themselves adopted healthy lifestyles (Rippe 2019, p. 967).

10. C According to Noffsinger, 2012, shared medical appointments are 'conservative individual medical visits in a supportive group setting where all can listen, interact, and learn'. These have been used as an adjunct clinical approach in several countries (Noffsinger 2012; Egger et al. 2015). They provide more time with the doctor, faster access to care, increased peer support, and greater opportunity for self-management (Egger et al. 2017, p. 58).

11. B The strongest and most compelling evidence is effectiveness of intensive therapeutic lifestyle change treatment (ITLC) because it produces the most dramatic treatment effects, just as higher dosing of pharmacological agents does. Conversely, few studies have been carried out on non-intensive lifestyle change programs. Their effectiveness is presumed based on published intensive therapeutic lifestyle change studies (Rippe 2019, p. 1019).

12. A Lifestyle Medicine is a distinct field of Medicine aimed at 'treating the cause' of most of our modern diseases with the strongest evidence-based modalities available. Since most modern diseases are caused by lifestyle, it stands to reason that lifestyle changes must be part of the cure. Although portions of Lifestyle Medicine (especially nutrition and physical activity) are included in other fields of medicine, lifestyle change is prescribed as the first-line and the most important therapy for disease treatment and reversal. Evidence-based medications and other modalities are used, but only to supplement changes in lifestyle (Kelly and Shull 2019, p. 15).

13. A Lifestyle Medicine is a distinct field of Medicine aimed at treating the root cause of most of our modern diseases. It is evidence-based and places a lot of emphasis on Behavioural Change. Integrative Medicine addresses the patient's whole person needs, employing a combination of experience-based complementary and alternative medicine methods with evidence-based conventional methods (Kelly and Shull 2019, p. 16).

14. C Functional Medicine focuses on the physiologic and biochemical functions of the body, investigating the balance and processes of cellular metabolism, digestive function, detoxification, and control of oxidative stress (Kelly and Shull 2019, p. 16).

15. D In Conventional Medicine, medications and surgical interventions are often the highest level of care and 'end' of treatment. In this disease-focused approach, patients are the recipients of care, while providers are considered responsible for care and outcomes (Kelly and Shull 2019, p. 16).

16. B Group consultations (the most common model used being Shared Medical Appointments) are fast gaining recognition as a viable adjunct clinical approach in the care of the patient. In the future, they are likely to become a standard procedure in clinical Lifestyle Medicine. Cognitive Behavioural Therapy is commonly used in the treatment protocols in Lifestyle Medicine. Lifestyle Medicine plays an important role in the prevention and treatment of many communicable diseases (Egger et al. 2017, p. 58).

17. D Preventive Medicine includes all aspects of morbidity and mortality prevention for the general public. It emphasizes population-based interventions that include immunizations, screening, and protection from bioterrorism (Kelly and Shull 2019, p. 16).

18. A Behavioural change is the foundational activity through which Lifestyle Medicine works. Health coaching involves assessing readiness for change, collaboratively establishing client goals, evaluating successful steps and self-limiting patterns, reassessing and modifying goals, articulating insights gained, and formulating post-coaching plan to sustain changes that promote health and wellness. The health coach does not change the lifestyle for the client, does not enforce behavioural change, and does not set goals for the client (Rippe 2019, p. 236).

19. **B** The following is the most appropriate technique in the behaviour change process:

In the early stages of change, use motivational interviewing

In the later stages of change, use cognitive behavioural therapy (CBT) technique

In all stages, use positive psychology

(Kelly and Shull 2019, p. 42)

20. **A** The field of Lifestyle Medicine envisages a world in which all physicians and allied health professionals have been trained and certified in evidence-based Lifestyle Medicine, integrating healthful behaviours into their own lives, while incorporating a Lifestyle Medicine-first approach to treating root causes of lifestyle-related diseases into their clinical practices. Therefore, ideally, physicians should serve as role-models in the practice of healthy personal behaviours. Leaders in LSM should promote healthy behaviours as foundational to medical care, disease prevention, and health promotion. Referrals to other specialists are sometimes indicated and must be done in a timely manner. Lifestyle management, helping patients manage and sustain healthy lifestyle practices, is a key competency for the physician in the practice of Lifestyle Medicine (Lianov and Johnson 2010; Tips Box 1.2).

21. **D** Assessment skills required by a physician in Lifestyle Medicine are varied. Physicians should assess patients and family readiness, willingness, and ability to make health behaviour changes. They should also perform a history and physical examination specific to patients' lifestyle-related health status (Kelly and Shull 2019, p. 26).

22. **C** The patients and their family's readiness and willingness is what is most required for a successful outcome in health coaching, much more than that of the community, employer, or support group (Kelly and Shull 2019, p. 26).

23. **A** Lifestyle Medicine treatment intensity has two components, namely intensity of contact hours and degree or extent of lifestyle changes made. Maximally effective intensive therapeutic lifestyle change generally maximizes both components (Rippe 2019, p. 1019).

24. **B** The intensive therapeutic lifestyle change (ITLC) produces the most dramatic treatment effects, just as higher dosing of pharmacological agents does. The ITLC maximizes Lifestyle Medicine treatment dosing to produce the induction phase needed to transform self-efficacy and enable the patient to sustain lifestyle change. For a lasting result, it will be preferable if an ITLC intervention is followed by therapeutic lifestyle change (TLC) treatment with the patient's primary care physician as follow-up is commonly the weak link that negates a very successful ITLC program (Rippe 2019, p. 1019).

TIPS BOX 1.2 | Lifestyle Medicine Competencies for Primary Care Physicians

Leadership
1) Promote healthy behaviours
2) Seek to practice, and create school, work, and home environments supporting, healthy behaviours.

Knowledge
3) Show knowing evidence on certain lifestyle changes improves patients' health outcomes
4) Describe ways physicians engage with patients/families can improve health behaviours

Assessment Skills
5) Assess social, psychological, and biological behaviours and resulting health outcomes
6) Assess readiness, willingness, and ability for health behavioural change
7) Perform lifestyle-specific history and physical examination, including lifestyle "vital signs" (diet, exercise, alcohol, smoking, BMI, sleep, stress, relationships), informing apt tests

Management Skills
8) Use recognized guidelines (e.g hypertension/quitting smoking) to help patients self-manage their lifestyles and choices.
9) Establish effective therapeutic relationships effecting and sustaining behaviour change with evidence-based counselling methods, tools and follow-up.
10) Collaborate with patients and their families to develop evidence-based, SMART action plans like lifestyle prescriptions.
11) Help patients manage/sustain healthy lifestyles and refer patients to appropriate healthcare professionals for lifestyle-related conditions

Use of Office and Community Support
12) Able to practice as an interdisciplinary healthcare team and support a team approach
13) Foster/use office routines supporting lifestyle medical care e.g decision support tools
14) Support quality improvement for lifestyle interventions with data
15) Refer appropriately in the community to support implementing healthy lifestyles

Adapted from *Lianov & Johnson,* 2010.

25. A The scientific foundation of the Erica Frank et al.'s 'Healthy Doctor = Healthy Patient' principle includes the following and more:

- North American physicians tend to live longer than their peers
- Physicians live longer because they have healthier habits (including as medical students) than their contemporaries
- Physicians and medical students with the healthiest habits are more likely to advise their patients about related preventive habits
- Counselling patients makes a difference in patients' habits and in their health

(Rippe 2019, p. 1039)

References

Barnard, N.D., Cohen, J., Jenkins, D.J. et al. (2009). A low-fat vegan diet and a conventional diabetes diet in the treatment of type 2 diabetes: a randomized, controlled, 74-wk clinical trial. *American Journal of Clinical Nutrition* 89 (5): 1588S–1596S. https://doi.org/10.3945/ajcn.2009.26736H.

Egger, G., Dixon, J., Meldrum, H., et al. (2015) Patients' and providers satisfaction with shared medical appointments. *Australian Family Physician* 44(9): 674–679. PMID: 26488050.

Egger, G., Binns, A., Rossner, S. et al. (2017). *Lifestyle Medicine: Lifestyle, the Environment and Preventive Medicine in Health and Disease*, 3e. Academic Press.

Frank, E. (2004) STUDENTJAMA. Physician health and patient care. JAMA 291(5):637. https://doi.org/10.1001/jama.291.5.637. PMID: 14762049.

Kelly, J. and Shull, J. (2019). *The Lifestyle Medicine Board Review Manual*, 2ee. American College of Lifestyle Medicine.

Lianov, L. and Johnson, M. (2012). Physician competencies for prescribing lifestyle medicine. *JAMA* 304(2):202-203. https://doi.org/10.1001/jama.2010.903. PMID: 20628134.

Noffsinger E.B. (2012). *The ABCs of group visits: an implementation manual for your practice*, 1e. Springer.

Ornish, D., Brown, S.E., Scherwitz, L.W. et al. (1990). Can lifestyle changes reverse coronary heart disease? The Lifestyle Heart Trial. *Lancet* 336 (8708): 129–133. https://doi.org/10.1016/0140-6736(90)91656-u. PMID: 1973470.

Rippe, J.M. (2019). *Lifestyle Medicine*, 3ee. CRC Press, Taylor & Francis Group.

Willett, W., Rockström, J., Loken, B. et al. (2019). Food in the Anthropocene: the EAT-Lancet Commission on healthy diets from sustainable food systems. *Lancet* 393 (10170): 447–492. https://doi.org/10.1016/S0140-6736(18)31788-4. Epub 2019 Jan 16. Erratum in: Lancet. 2019 Feb 9;393(10171):530. Erratum in: Lancet. 2019 Jun 29;393(10191):2590. Erratum in: Lancet. 2020 Feb 1;395(10221):338. Erratum in: Lancet. 2020 Oct 3;396(10256):e56. PMID: 30660336.

CHAPTER 2

Fundamentals of Health Behaviour Change

Introduction

Behaviour change is the mainstay in the delivery of lifestyle medicine interventions. It is important that clinicians are familiar with behaviour change techniques that foster self-efficacy and cultivate a therapeutic relationship to empower the change process. Knowledge of different theories is essential. Practising the different techniques with patients will enable clinicians to become proficient in them. The emphasis is on listening rather than informing the patient, motivating rather than convincing the patient, and collaborating with the patient rather than directing the patient.

This chapter tests the candidate's knowledge of health behaviour, change theories, and how they can be applied in practice to help patients maintain healthy behaviour. It tests the candidate's ability to apply motivational interviewing, cognitive behaviour therapy, and positive psychology techniques to the behaviour change process.

1. Which of the following best describes the 'action' stage of the Transtheoretical Model of health behaviour?

    a. The patient has been making changes within the last six months

    b. The doctor assists with plans on specific changes

    c. The patient intends to make changes within six months

    d. The patient intends to make some changes within one month

Lifestyle Medicine: Essential MCQs for Certification in Lifestyle Medicine, First Edition.
Ifeoma Monye, Adaeze Ifezulike, Karen Adamson and Fraser Birrell.
© 2022 John Wiley & Sons Ltd. Published 2022 by John Wiley & Sons Ltd.

2. Which of the following options best describes the Health Belief Model (HBM) of behaviour change theory?

    a. Different interventions should be used at different stages of behaviour change

    b. Governmental policies lead to health behaviour change

    c. Self-efficacy and perceived susceptibility to health threat leads to behavior change

    d. Social reinforcement leads to a patient maintaining a healthy behaviour

3. Which of the following most appropriately describes the levels of influence on health behavior change?

    a. Community factors and social network

    b. Intrapersonal, interpersonal, and institutional factors

    c. Introspective factors, beliefs, and personality

    d. Public rules, regulations, and policies

4. A 48-year-old woman attends for a review of her asthma and when you mention her BMI of 40 kg/m², she informs you that she has been thinking of buying an exercise bike for her birthday in two months' time and becoming more active. What stage of health behaviour change does this best describe?

    a. Action stage

    b. Contemplation stage

    c. Precontemplation stage

    d. Preparation stage

5. Which of the following management options will be most appropriate for a person on the precontemplation stage?

    a. Discuss health risks and benefits of a healthy lifestyle

    b. Discuss mindfulness-based stress reduction

    c. Personalize their health risk based on medical history

    d. Referral to a dietician for meal planning

6. The action stage of health behaviour change is best characterized by which of the following?

    a. The doctor gives a personalized analysis of risk based on the patient's history

    b. The doctor maps out an action plan for the patient to endorse

    c. The patient has been making specific health modifications within the past six months

    d. The patient is encouraged to list out all the possible barriers to making progress

7. Which of the following would be the best practice in facilitating health behaviour changes?

    a. Aim to document a behaviour change plan in every patient's health records every year

    b. Ensure that every patient leaves with a clear relapse plan

c. Making available a readiness assessment for patients to complete in advance in the waiting room

d. Review the patient's completed readiness assessment form to prioritize lifestyle areas you want the patient to change

8. A health behaviour change theory that best explains the reciprocal influence of personal factors, environmental factors, and the health behaviour on the individual is:

a. Health Review Model

b. Social Learning (Cognitive) Theory

c. Theory of Reasonable Behaviour

d. Theory of Socially Accepted Behaviour

9. Key behaviour theories have several similarities. Which of these options best describes the common features?

a. Environmental influence, e.g. socially accepted norms guarantee behaviours

b. Motivation and beliefs about risk and benefits of the health behaviour underpin change

c. One's confidence in ability to complete the behaviour change is key

d. Regular self-criticism and reflection aids in behaviour

10. Which of these options is the most appropriate skill in facilitating sustainable behaviour changes at the early stages?

a. Cognitive behaviour techniques

b. Motivational interviewing

c. Positive psychology

d. Reframing non-productive thinking

11. Which of these options best represents the precontemplation stage of behaviour change?

a. I am not thinking about making a change at all

b. I have started a change within the last six months

c. I am thinking of making a change within the next six months

d. I have been making a change for more than six months

12. Which of the following is the most appropriate management in stage-matched interventions?

a. Offer an intervention that is acceptable to majority of patients

b. Offer an intervention that is tailored to the patient's readiness for a specific action

c. Offer an intervention that is used by all patients

d. Offer an intervention that the patient has failed before so he can perfect it

13. Which of these options best represents the process in Stage-Matched Interventions?
    a. Family support should not be solicited as this encourages dependence
    b. It is important that the patient completes every item at each stage
    c. The degree of readiness is not an important factor
    d. The doctor aims to help the patient move from one stage of readiness to the next

14. Thomas is considering becoming more active within the next 30 days to tackle his obesity. Which of these will be the most appropriate action?
    a. Check his level of confidence in his ability to carry out his plans
    b. Discuss health risk associated with specific behaviour
    c. Give him a lifestyle prescription
    d. Use CBT to reframe unhealthy thought patterns

15. You are worried that Gabriel still smokes heavily despite his COPD. However, he tells you categorically that he is not willing to give up this habit. Which of these is the most appropriate action for his stage of readiness?
    a. You ask the patient to write down his unwillingness to change despite medical advice
    b. You provide a general healthy lifestyle advice
    c. You try some CBT techniques to see if you might change his mind
    d. You try to problem-solve his barriers to stopping smoking

16. Mike tells you that he is already making a change to tackle his unhealthy eating habits. Which of these is the most appropriate next step in his management?
    a. Develop a relapse prevention plan if he has been making the change for three months
    b. Discuss health risks associated with his unhealthy eating habit
    c. Give him an action plan if he is not meeting his goal yet
    d. Use CBT to reframe any unhealthy thought patterns

17. Which of the following best describes the stages of readiness?
    a. CBT methods work best when started early
    b. Patients need one month of coaching to complete each stage
    c. Positive psychology is counterproductive at the beginning stage
    d. The goal is to move the patient from his current level of readiness to the next stage

18. Which of the following would be most appropriate to include in Health Behaviour Change Readiness tool which a patient could fill while in the waiting room?
    a. An assessment of the patient's confidence that he can improve his nutrition
    b. An assessment of the patient's marital status and political inclination

  c. An assessment of the patient's perceived importance of lifestyle medicine

  d. An assessment of the patient's perceived importance of their intellectual abilities

19. Readiness for a change in health behaviour is best determined by which of the following?

  a. The doctor's track record skill of motivational interviewing

  b. The government's motivations for recommending the change

  c. The importance the society attaches to the change

  d. The patient's confidence level in making the change

20. Which of these is the most appropriate feature of a health behaviour change assessment tool?

  a. Patient's cultural background

  b. Patient's literacy level

  c. Patient's marital status

  d. Patient's responses prioritize areas for discussion

21. To facilitate the 'Coach' mindset of the Physician, which of the following is the most appropriate recommendation?

  a. Be open and compassionate

  b. Compel the patient to write his goals down

  c. Offer a congratulatory hug to patients for each goal achieved

  d. Send a copy of his action plan to his spouse for accountability

22. Which one of these was best demonstrated in the study by Hojat published in the Academic Medicine 2011 on Provider–Patient relationship and illustrated that patients valued empathy from their physician?

  a. Improved HbA1c control

  b. Improved literacy levels

  c. Improved social skills

  d. Improved spousal engagement

23. Which statement best summarizes the findings of the study on Provider–Patient relationship Cochrane systematic review (Dwamena et al. 2012)?

  a. 10-hour training of providers on attentiveness and empathy did not yield any positive effect on the consultation process

  b. 10-hour training on empathy skills achieved the same result as longer training

  c. Longer training was favoured by most physicians

  d. The skills had a negligible effect on the consultation process

24. Which of the following best describes key component of good Patient–Provider relationship?

    a. Empathetically dwelling on the patient's negative feelings

    b. Identifying the patient's concerns and applying positive psychology

    c. Instructive criticism and goal setting

    d. Listening carefully and encouraging self-criticism

25. Which of these approaches is best used in applying the Physician 'Coach' Mindset?

    a. Discourage family involvement as the patient should not be distracted

    b. Encourage patients to take careful note of their weaknesses

    c. Explain that obstacles and setbacks on the behaviour change path signals' poor outcome

    d. Share personal examples where disclosure would support the patient

26. Which of these sets of approaches are most appropriate in the 5 As approach to health behaviour counselling?

    a. Advise, agree, approach

    b. Arrange, amend, acknowledge

    c. Assess, advise, agree

    d. Assist, amend, arrange

27. Which one of these is the most appropriate statement about the 5 As approach to health counselling?

    a. Confrontational approach works well in stubborn patients

    b. It can be used as a brief health behaviour counselling

    c. Motivational speeches are necessary to suppress the patient's opposition to change

    d. Positive psychology should be done by trained psychologists

28. Facilitating behaviour change is best achieved by which of the following?

    a. Cognitive behaviour techniques at earlier stages of change

    b. Motivational interviewing at the later stages of change

    c. Positive psychology at all stages

    d. Writing down treatment goals

29. It is most appropriate during Motivational Interviewing to do which of the following?

    a. Develop discrepancy between where the patient is and what the patient wants

    b. Ensure that the physician sits on the green coaching chair

    c. Roll with repentance by remaining non-judgemental

    d. Support self-criticism of the patient's ability to succeed

30. Motivational Interviewing techniques are useful when discussing weight and lifestyle interventions with patients. It's most helpful to do which of the following?

    a. Acknowledge the patient's prior efforts

    b. Emphasize that the cause of obesity is simply overeating

    c. Ensure that obese patients all line up to check their weight in the waiting room

    d. Realize that most obese people have never attempted to lose weight

31. Which of these patterns most represents a type of non-productive thinking harmful to the patient?

    a. All or nothing thinking

    b. Catastrophe avoiding

    c. Mind mapping

    d. Undergeneralization

32. Which of these most suitably describes a feature of unproductive thinking useful to identify in Cognitive Behavioural Therapy (CBT)?

    a. Catastrophe avoiding

    b. Happiness acting

    c. 'Should' and 'must' statements

    d. Undergeneralization

33. Which one of these options best explains how Cognitive Behavioural Therapy (CBT) helps patients?

    a. Decrease awareness of their upsetting emotions

    b. Discourage parental input

    c. Mask underlying beliefs that can interfere with behaviour change

    d. Reframe thoughts to support behaviour change

34. Cognitive Behavioural Therapy (CBT) is best used in what stages of change?

    a. Contemplation and precontemplation stages

    b. Maintenance and precontemplation stages

    c. Precontemplation and action stages

    d. Preparation and action stages

35. Which of these best explains the role of the clinician during the clinic visit?

    a. Encourage more realistic interpretations of thoughts

    b. Facilitate the patient in examining evidence for and against his thoughts

    c. Insistence on homework assignments for the patient to practise new thinking strategies

    d. Monitor and explore all thoughts that the patient has

36. Which of the following is the most accurate interpretation of the acronym ABCD in the ABCD method of identifying underlying beliefs that can interfere with behaviour change?

    a. Assess the patient's readiness for change

    b. Berate self about what has occurred

    c. Consequences of those beliefs should be explored

    d. Deal with those beliefs

37. Which of the following is the best description of a successful relapse prevention plan?

    a. Focusing on self-criticism when you notice a lapse

    b. Identifying people to blame for a lapse

    c. Knowing what to do when a lapse occurs

    d. Taking steps to write down your action plan

38. Which of the following is a key step in Positive Psychology?

    a. Building on dreams

    b. Discouraging thoughts

    c. Encouraging criticism

    d. Reinforcing self-efficacy

39. Which of the following is the best description of the important role the patient's social and environmental factors play in their health behaviour change?

    a. Can help support accountability

    b. Can have a negative influence due to scrutiny

    c. Should ideally be faith-based

    d. Should never be electronic social networks due to distractions

40. Which of the following is the most effective at undermining health behaviour change?

    a. Faith-based groups

    b. Family and friends

    c. Peer modelling strategies

    d. Poor goal setting

41. Positive relationships can help support the patient's health journey by encouraging which of the following?

    a. Self-accounting

    b. Self-autonomy

  c. Self-criticism

  d. Self-effacing

42. Which of the following is the most appropriate way for care providers to empower patients?

  a. Encouraging dependency on family

  b. Providing monetary support

  c. Providing social entertainment

  d. Signposting to environmental and social support

43. Which of the following is a key feature of poor counselling techniques on health behaviour change?

  a. Encouraging introspection and focus on areas of weakness

  b. Encouraging the involvement of family members in action plans

  c. Guiding the patient to do a social support analysis

  d. Offer stage-matched intervention at every visit

44. 52-year-old Sue has been found to have high cholesterol of 7.2 mmol/l. She says she hates vegetables and would not ever eat them. She is already considering registering with a gym to increase her physical activity but is concerned her bad knee may not allow her exercise much.

 On the advice of a friend, she has bought a cookery book to explore healthy meals that do not include vegetables. What is the best course of action to facilitate her health behaviour change journey?

  a. Cognitive Behavioural Therapy (CBT) to address her concern that her knee would be a limiting factor

  b. Cognitive Behavioural Therapy (CBT) to counter her hatred of vegetables

  c. Motivational interviewing to address her plans of registering with a gym

  d. Motivational interviewing to address her use of the cookery book

45. Lucy has a blood pressure of 173/92. She is adamant that she will not take medication. She is keen to try lifestyle changes and is already cooking with less salt and adding garlic to her meals. She refuses to go for a walk as she is afraid of the youngsters hanging about the street corners and her husband is always too tired to come walking with her.

 What is the best course of action to address her concerns?

  a. Cognitive Behavioural Therapy (CBT) to explore her mindset about taking medication

  b. Motivational Interviewing to address her fear of youngsters in the street

  c. Motivational Interviewing to address the perceived limiting effect that her husband's tiredness is having on her health

  d. Positive psychology to affirm what she is already doing with her meals

46. Which of the following is the most appropriate step in effective consultation during Action Planning?

    a. Address the patient's questions about his diagnosis

    b. Confront the patient on his lack of progress

    c. Summarize the patient's comments to show how negative he is

    d. The doctor sets goals for patients to facilitate their behaviour change

47. In the precontemplation stage of health behaviour change, it is most appropriate to do which of the following?

    a. Ask the patient to identify the major obstacle to completing goal and strategy to overcome it

    b. Elicit the patient's level of confidence in achieving a specific goal (1–10 with 10 being extremely confident)

    c. Ensure goals are specific

    d. Give general advice on benefits of leading a healthy lifestyle

48. Action plans are lifestyle prescriptions tailored to the individual patient. Which of these is most appropriate to consider when drawing up action plans?

    a. Ability

    b. Family

    c. Neighbourhood

    d. Social connections

49. Lifestyle prescriptions are best based on which of the following?

    a. Current level of activity

    b. May be adjusted as the patient's situation changes

    c. The patient's readiness for change

    d. Scientific evidence

50. Which of the following is best considered in relapse prevention plans?

    a. Develop plan at the precontemplation stage

    b. Fixed to ensure stability

    c. Rechecked with the patient as life situations change

    d. Should not be planned in anticipation of a relapse

51. At which of these points is Cognitive Behavioural Therapy (CBT) most useful?

    a. At the precontemplation stage of change

    b. The patient is experiencing feelings of courage

    c. The patient is feeling out of control

    d. When the patient is succeeding with his goals to prevent him from getting too comfortable

52. Which of these most accurately describes relapse?

a. Relapse is a sustained period when an action plan is not followed

b. Relapse is easier to address before it becomes a habit

c. Relapse is more likely to occur if an action plan is written down

d. Relapse needs to be addressed as a continuation of the previous action plan

53. Which of these most accurately describes lapse?

a. Lapse is a short period when an action plan was not followed

b. Lapse is more likely to occur if an action plan is written down

c. It can take less energy to re-start an action plan if allowed to lapse for a long time

d. It is easier to deal with a lapse by allowing some time to pass before revisiting the issue

54. Which of the following is the most appropriate to address in a relapse prevention plan?

a. Disclosing the frequency of lapse occurrence in the population

b. The patient identifying when a lapse is likely to occur and what to do then

c. What occupation predisposes the patient to lapses

d. What the patient's neighbours frequently engage in that can cause a lapse

55. Which of these is the most appropriate self-management strategies for lapse prevention?

a. Digital and live exploration of triggers

b. Frequent exposure to lapse triggers

c. Making use of the friends' recommended social media sites

d. Support with digital self-help apps

56. Danny started smoking again after three months of abstinence. He now wants to quit smoking again. Which of these is the most appropriate advice for him?

a. Create a backup plan at the time of any relapse to enable you stay on track.

b. Encourage a significant other to help remind you of your action plan when they notice a lapse

c. Frequent exposure to your smoking buddies to develop tolerance

d. Reach out to your care provider when you find yourself off action plan for more than a few months

57. As a care provider, your most appropriate next step in facilitating your client's action plan is to:

a. Emphasize the importance of a verbal action plan

b. Ensure action plans are completed based on readiness for appropriate behaviour change

c. Keep a copy of the action plan in the medical archives

d. Review action plans every year

58. Which one of these is best avoided by the coach during follow-up visits?

a. Confront the patient's lack of progress

b. Congratulate the patient on the progress made

c. Discuss barriers and develop solutions

d. Discuss the progress made by the patient

59. Which of the following is best avoided during follow-up?

a. Failures should be discussed first

b. Have a patient's action plan in front of you

c. Reflect back what the patient has reported to show an understanding

d. Successes should be discussed first

60. Lifestyle prescriptions are best described by which of the following?

a. Evidence-based

b. Specific to the patient's peculiar health issue

c. Tailored to the patient's abilities

d. The same as action plans

61. What is the next best step using motivational interviewing techniques in a patient who wants his chest to get better but does not want to stop smoking?

a. The interviewer needs to discuss an action plan with the patient

b. The interviewer should develop discrepancy between where the patient is and what he wants

c. The interviewer should withhold empathy to demonstrate the seriousness of the issue

d. The patient's resistance is a cue to the interviewer to insist on a quit attempt

62. Which of the following statements most appropriately describes cognitive behavioural techniques?

a. It assists with deeper understanding of underlying challenges

b. It is the counsellor's job to generate the solutions as the expert

c. Patient ambivalence is accepted as a natural part of change process

d. Patient resistance is decreased using non-confrontational methods

Answers

1. A In the Action stage of behaviour change, the person has been making a change in the last six months (Hashemzadeh et al. 2019; Selçuk-Tosun and Zinci, 2019).

2. C Governmental policies do not play a key role in the Health Belief Model. The model explains that before one will seek preventative measures, he must first believe there is a threat to his health and a preventative measure that is accessible and low risk that will enable him to avoid the health threat (Stokols and Zmuidzinas 2000; LaMorte 2018; Sheppard and Thomas 2020).

3. B Intrapersonal factors like one's knowledge, attitudes, beliefs, and personality influence their health behaviour in addition to other influences like interpersonal factors, community factors, and public policies (LaMorte 2018; Beauchamp et al. 2019).

4. B Any change being contemplated within six months is at the contemplation stage (Hashemzadeh et al. 2019; Selçuk-Tosun and Zincir 2019).

5. A For a person at the precontemplation stage, you can only discuss the health benefits of a healthy lifestyle in general terms (Hashemzadeh et al. 2019; Selçuk-Tosun and Zincir 2019).

6. C The person at the action stage has been making a change within the past six months (Hashemzadeh et al. 2019; Selçuk-Tosun and Zincir 2019).

7. C Making available a readiness assessment for patients to complete in advance in the waiting room, documenting behaviour change plan in every patient's health records at each visit and reviewing the patient's completed readiness assessment form to prioritize lifestyle areas which the patient is most ready to address are tips a clinician could use to facilitate health behaviour change (Kelly and Shull 2019, p. 41; Tips Box 2.1).

TIPS BOX 2.1 | Factors Influencing Health Behaviour

A person's health behaviour is influenced by:

a. Intrapersonal factors such as his knowledge, attitude, beliefs, and personality

b. Interpersonal factors such as influence of peers, health providers, friends, and family

c. Institutional factors such as the community norms and public policies

Source: Kelly and Shull (2019).

8. B Social Learning theory explains 'reciprocal determinism' in which the patient, the behaviour, and the environment all influence each other (Chen et al. 2015; Beauchamp et al. 2019).

9. B Self-efficacy as well as motivation, beliefs about risks and benefits of change and Social Norms are things key behaviour theories have in common (Kelly and Shull 2019, p. 40).

10. B Positive psychology, Motivational Interviewing, and Cognitive Behaviour Techniques are useful skills in facilitating the behaviour change process. Motivational Interviewing is most helpful at the early stages of change (Miller and Rollnick 2012; Soderlund 2018).

11. A In the precontemplation stage, the patient is not thinking about making a change at all now or within the next six months (Hashemzadeh et al. 2019; Selçuk-Tosun and Zincir 2019).

12. B Stage-matched interventions must be appropriate to the person's readiness to change to encourage adherence (Crespo et al. 2019; Hashemzadeh et al. 2019; Selçuk-Tosun and Zincir 2019; Tips Box 2.2).

13. D Ideally, the plan for change should be dictated by the patient. However, the doctor acts as a coach to facilitate this. Family support, if available and positive, can help facilitate changes in health behaviour (Kelly and Shull 2019, p. 42).

14. A Assessing readiness and confidence levels are appropriate. CBT is used at later stages of change. Lifestyle prescriptions are not specific to each patient and general advice is best used at the precontemplation stage which this person has already passed (Kelly and Shull 2019, p. 41).

15. B This is the precontemplation stage and it will be appropriate to raise the issue at another consultation as the patient may have changed his mind. Exploring his health beliefs and providing general healthy lifestyle advice are appropriate (DiClemente et al. 1991; Stewart and Fox 2011; Crespo et al. 2019).

TIPS BOX 2.2 | Stages of Change

Techniques such as Motivational Interviewing, Cognitive Behavioural Therapy (CBT), and Positive Psychology are used to assist patients in the behaviour change process:

a. In the early stages of change (precontemplation and contemplation stages), Motivational Interviewing is helpful

b. In the preparation, action, and maintenance stages, CBT is most useful

c. All stages of change can benefit from Positive Psychology

Sources: Hashemzadeh et al. (2019) and Selçuk-Tosun and Zincir (2019).

16. D In a person who is already making changes, CBT skills are useful in addressing any unhelpful thought patterns (Keles and Idsoe 2018; Trifu et al., 2019; Beck 2020).

17. D Positive psychology is used at all stages while Motivational Interviewing methods come in handy in the early stages (Wong 2011; Fredrickson and Joiner 2018).

18. A An assessment of the patient's confidence in the key areas of lifestyle change such as stress management, nutrition, and physical activity is helpful and forms the basis of the subsequent discussion when they go in to see the clinician (Kelly and Shull 2019, p. 41).

19. D The person's confidence in managing the change is a key factor in determining their ability to accomplish the goal (Bandura 2010; Ha et al. 2018).

20. D A healthcare provider uses the health assessment tool to prioritize areas for discussion as highlighted by the patient's responses in the questionnaire (Kelly and Shull 2019, p. 41).

21. A A hug may be unprofessional, and the patients should be encouraged, not compelled, to write down their goals (Hicks and McCracken 2009; Frates and Bonnet 2016).

22. A Better HbA1c control is the correct study outcome in the list. The study demonstrated that empathy is a clinically important factor in patient outcomes (Hojat et al. 2011).

23. B 10-hour training on empathy skills achieved the same result as longer training and had a positive effect on the consultation (Lewin et al. 2001; Dwamena et al. 2012; Boissy et al. 2016).

24. B While the other options may have a role to play, identifying the patient's concerns and applying positive psychology are key aspects of a successful consultation (Boissy et al. 2016; Fredrickson and Joiner 2018).

25. D Sharing personal examples where disclosure would support a patient's journey is a useful skill in coaching (Kelly and Shull 2019, p. 53).

26. C The 5 As approach to health behaviour counselling are Assess, Advise, Agree, Assist, and Arrange follow-up (Whitlock et al. 2002; Jay et al. 2010).

27. B The 5 As approach can be used as a brief health behaviour counselling or as part of longer ongoing counselling (Whitlock et al. 2002; Jay et al. 2010; Stewart and Fox 2011).

28. C While writing down treatment plans is useful, this is not appropriate in the precontemplation stage, whereas positive psychology is important at every stage (Alexandrova 2017; Fredrickson and Joiner 2018).

29. A The ability to develop discrepancy between where the patient is and what the patient wants is a key skill in motivational interviewing. The other key features are expressing empathy, rolling with resistance, and supporting self-efficacy (Miller and Rollnick 2012; Soderlund 2018; Tolchin et al. 2019).

30. **A** The cause of obesity is complex. It is a sensitive topic, and it is helpful to check the patient's weight in private (Kelly and Shull 2019, p. 55).

31. **A** All or nothing thinking is unproductive. The other options are not recognized thinking patterns (Trifu et al. 2019; Beck 2020).

32. **C** 'Should' and 'must' statements are features of unproductive thinking (Trifu et al. 2019; Beck 2020).

33. **D** Cognitive Behavioural Therapy (CBT) helps patients unmask underlying beliefs that affect behaviour change. Positive parental input is encouraged. Reframing thoughts to support behaviour change is important (Trifu et al. 2019; Beck 2020).

34. **D** Cognitive Behavioural Therapy (CBT) is best used in preparation, action, and maintenance stages (Kelly and Shull 2019, p. 42).

35. **A** Encouraging more realistic interpretations of thoughts in patients is an important CBT skill (Trifu et al. 2019; Beck 2020).

36. **C** Exploring the consequences of one's beliefs is one of the ABCD methods of identifying underlying beliefs that can interfere with behaviour change. A refers to the action or event that has occurred, B is the belief one has about what occurred, and D encourages the patient to dispute unhealthy beliefs. C is consequences of those beliefs should be explored. (Sarracino et al. 2017; Kelly and Shull 2019, p. 43; Tips Box 2.3).

37. **C** A successful relapse prevention plan involves knowing what to do when a lapse occurs (Larimer et al. 1999; Kelly and Shull 2019, p. 50).

38. **D** A key step in Positive Psychology is the promotion of self-efficacy in patients. Positive psychology aims to build a patient's confidence by emphasizing their current skills, abilities, and positive actions. It enhances resilience and helps undo negative feelings (Wong 2011; Fredrickson and Joiner 2018).

TIPS BOX 2.3 | ABCD Method of Behavioural Change

Unhelpful beliefs can interfere with the behaviour change process. Using the ABCD method can help identify these underlying beliefs:

   a. What ACTION occurred?
   b. What BELIEFS do you have about what occurred?
   c. What are the CONSEQUENCES of those beliefs?
   d. Attempt to DISPUTE those beliefs that are unhealthy

Sources: Sarracino et al. (2017) and Kelly and Shull (2019).

39. A A patient's social and environmental factors can help support accountability, need not be faith-based, and can involve judicious use of electronic social support sites (Kelly and Shull 2019, p. 44).

40. D Goal setting using the SMART format can help the patient stay on track (Kelly and Shull 2019, p. 47).

41. B Positive relationships with significant others can help support self-autonomy (Bandura 2010; Ha et al. 2018).

42. D Providing monetary support, unnecessary social entertainment, and encouraging reliance on family undermine the patient's self-efficacy and are not a usual part of the physician's professional input (Bandura 2010; Ha et al. 2018).

43. A Excessive focus on areas of weakness and negative introspection where patients turn against themselves can be a hindrance to behaviour change (Trifu et al. 2019; Beck 2020).

44. A Cognitive Behavioural Therapy (CBT) is best used in preparation, action, and maintenance stages. She is already prepared to use the gym but is worried her knee will limit her ability. CBT techniques can help her reframe this limiting thought by realizing she can start gently and do more as time goes on (Fredrickson and Joiner 2018; Soderlund 2018).

45. D Positive psychology to affirm what she is already doing with her meals is the best course of action at this stage (Fredrickson and Joiner 2018; Crespo et al. 2019).

46. A Addressing a patient's ideas, concerns, and expectations (ICE) is a good practice. Summarizing shows good listening and understanding abilities (Miller 2018; Ng and Luk 2019).

47. D Goal setting is not appropriate in the precontemplation stage. General advice on benefits of leading a healthy lifestyle should be given (Miller and Rollnick 2012; Kelly and Shull 2019, p. 45).

48. A Action plans are based on the patient's ability, readiness, and confidence (Kelly and Shull 2019, p. 45).

49. D Lifestyle prescriptions are based on scientific evidence (Kelly and Shull 2019, p. 45).

50. C It is a good practice to have a relapse prevention plan constructed for each behaviour change and the plan reviewed as the patient's life circumstances change (Larimer et al. 1999; Kelly and Shull 2019, p. 50).

51. C CBT assists with problem solving and deeper understanding of underlying challenges (Trifu et al. 2019; Beck 2020).

52. A A relapse is a sustained period when an action plan is not followed (Larimer et al. 1999; Witkiewitz and Marlatt 2004).

53. A A lapse is a short period when an action plan was not followed (Larimer et al. 1999; Witkiewitz and Marlatt 2004).

54. **B**   A relapse prevention plan should explore triggers for lapses such as when, under what circumstances, with whom, and who to turn to during a relapse (Kelly and Shull 2019, p. 50).

55. **D**   Support with digital self-help apps (Kelly and Shull 2019, p. 46).

56. **B**   Encouraging a significant other to help remind you of your action plan when they notice a lapse is the most appropriate advice (Kelly and Shull 2019, p. 50).

57. **B**   Ensure action plans are completed based on readiness for appropriate behaviour change. Action plans should be written and reviewed at each visit (Kelly and Shull 2019, p. 48).

58. **A**   The confronting patient should be avoided and positive psychology applied instead (Wong 2011; Fredrickson and Joiner 2018).

59. **A**   Successes, not failures, should be discussed first (Wong 2011; Fredrickson and Joiner 2018).

60. **A**   Lifestyle prescriptions are based on scientific evidence and the patient's medical condition (Lianov and Johnson 2010; Kelly and Shull 2019, p. 45).

61. **B**   The interviewer should develop a discrepancy between where the patient is and what he wants (Yakovenko et al. 2015; Soderlund 2018; Tolchin et al. 2019).

62. **A**   CBT assists with a deeper understanding of the underlying challenges. The other options describe motivational interviewing techniques (Trifu et al. 2019; Beck 2020).

References

Alexandrova, A. (2017). *A Philosophy for the Science of Well-being*. Oxford University Press.

Bandura, A. (2010). Self-efficacy. In: *The Corsini Encyclopaedia of Psychology*, 1–3. Wiley Online Library.

Beauchamp, M.R., Crawford, K.L., and Jackson, B. (2019). Social cognitive theory and physical activity: Mechanisms of behaviour change, critique, and legacy. *Psychology of Sport and Exercise* 42: 110–117.

Beck, J.S. (2020). *Cognitive Behaviour Therapy: Basics and Beyond*. Guilford Publications.

Boissy, A., Windover, A.K., Bokar, D. et al. (2016). Communication skills training for physicians improves patient satisfaction. *Journal of General Internal Medicine* 31 (7): 755–761.

Chen, M.F., Wang, R.H., and Hung, S.L. (2015). Predicting health-promoting self-care behaviours in people with pre-diabetes by applying Bandura social learning theory. *Applied Nursing Research* 28 (4): 299–304.

Crespo, F.S., Jaén-Moreno, M.J., Gutiérrez-Rojas, L. et al. (2019). "Readiness to change" predicts efficacy of reduction among smokers with severe mental illness. *European Addiction Research* 25 (5): 256–262.

DiClemente, C.C., Prochaska, J.O., Fairhurst, S.K. et al. (1991). The process of smoking cessation: an analysis of precontemplation, contemplation, and preparation stages of change. *Journal of Consulting and Clinical Psychology* 59 (2): 295.

Dwamena, F., Holmes-Rovner, M., Gaulden, C.M. et al. (2012). Interventions for providers to promote a patient-centred approach in clinical consultations. *Cochrane Database of Systematic Review* 12: CD003267. https://doi.org/10.1002/14651858.CD003267.pub2. PMID: 23235595.

Frates, E.P. and Bonnet, J. (2016). Collaboration and negotiation: the key to therapeutic lifestyle change. *American Journal of Lifestyle Medicine* 10 (5): L302–L312.

Fredrickson, B.L. and Joiner, T. (2018). Reflections on positive emotions and upward spirals. *Perspectives on Psychological Science* 13 (2): 194–199.

Ha, F.J., Hare, D.L., Cameron, J.D., and Toukhsati, S.R. (2018). Heart failure and exercise: a narrative review of the role of self-efficacy. *Heart, Lung and Circulation* 27 (1): 22–27.

Hashemzadeh, M., Rahimi, A., Zare-Farashbandi, F. et al. (2019). Transtheoretical model of health behavioural change: a systematic review. *Iranian Journal of Nursing and Midwifery Research* 24 (2): 83.

Hicks, R. and McCracken, J. (2009). Mentoring vs. coaching-do you know the difference? *Physician Executive* 35 (4): 71–73.

Hojat, M., Louis, D.Z., Markham, F.W. et al. (2011). Physicians' empathy and clinical outcomes for diabetic patients. *Academic Medicine* 86 (3): 359–364.

Jay, M., Gillespie, C., Schlair, S. et al. (2010). Physicians' use of the 5As in counseling obese patients: is the quality of counseling associated with patients' motivation and intention to lose weight? *BMC Health Services Research* 10 (1): 159.

Keles, S. and Idsoe, T. (2018). A meta-analysis of group cognitive behavioural therapy (CBT) interventions for adolescents with depression. *Journal of Adolescence* 67: 129–139.

Kelly, J. and Shull, J. (2019). *Foundations of Lifestyle Medicine: Lifestyle Medicine Board Review Manual*, 2ee, 39–61. American College of Lifestyle Medicine.

LaMorte, W.W. (2018). *Behavioural Change Models: The Health Belief Model*. Boston University, School of Public Health.

Larimer, M.E., Palmer, R.S., and Marlatt, G.A. (1999). Relapse prevention: an overview of Marlatt's cognitive-behavioural model. *Alcohol Research & Health* 23 (2): 151.

Lewin, S., Skea, Z., Entwistle, V.A. et al. (2001). Interventions for providers to promote a patient-centred approach in clinical consultations. *Cochrane Database of Systematic Reviews* 12: CD003267. https://doi.org/10.1002/14651858.CD003267. PMID: 11687181.

Lianov, L. and Johnson, M. (2010). Physician competencies for prescribing lifestyle medicine. *JAMA* 304 (2): 202–203. https://doi.org/10.1001/jama.2010.903.

Miller, A. (2018). A patient expectation and satisfaction survey with regards to exercise prescription from their osteopathic manual practitioner. *International Journal of Whole Person Care* 5 (1) https://doi.org/10.26443/ijwpc.v5i1.177.

Miller, W.R. and Rollnick, S. (2012). *Motivational Interviewing: Helping people change*. Guilford press.

Ng, J.H. and Luk, B.H. (2019). Patient satisfaction: concept analysis in the healthcare context. *Patient Education and Counseling* 102 (4): 790–796.

Sarracino, D., Dimaggio, G., Ibrahim, R. et al. (2017). When REBT goes difficult: applying ABC-DEF to personality disorders. *Journal of Rational-Emotive & Cognitive-Behaviour Therapy* 35 (3): 278–295.

Selçuk-Tosun, A. and Zincir, H. (2019). The effect of a transtheoretical model–based motivational interview on self-efficacy, metabolic control, and health behaviour in adults with type 2 diabetes mellitus: A randomized controlled trial. *International Journal of Nursing Practice* 25 (4): e12742.

Sheppard, J. and Thomas, C.B. (2020). Community pharmacists and communication in the time of COVID-19: applying the health belief model. Research in Social and Administrative Pharmacy.

Soderlund, P.D. (2018). Effectiveness of motivational interviewing for improving physical activity self-management for adults with type 2 diabetes: a review. *Chronic Illness* 14 (1): 54–68.

Stewart, E.E. and Fox, C.H. (2011). Encouraging patients to change unhealthy behaviours with motivational interviewing. *Family Practice Management* 18 (3): 21. https://www.aafp.org/dam/AAFP/documents/patient_care/nrn/motivinterview2.pdf.

Stokols, D. and Zmuidzinas, M. (2000). Modelling and managing change in. Person-environment psychology: new directions and perspectives, p. 267.

Tolchin, B., Baslet, G., Suzuki, J. et al. (2019). Randomized controlled trial of motivational interviewing for psychogenic nonepileptic seizures. *Epilepsia* 60 (5): 986–995.

Trifu, S., Popescu, A., and Dragoi, A.M. (2019). The fight of patient with paranoid Schizophrenia disorder with his the psychiatric diagnosis: a game of "everything or nothing". *International Journal of Research-GRANTHAALAYAH* 7 (11): 240–248.

Whitlock, E.P., Orleans, C.T., Pender, N., and Allan, J. (2002). Evaluating primary care behavioural counseling interventions: an evidence-based approach. *American Journal of Preventive Medicine* 22 (4): 267–284.

Witkiewitz, K. and Marlatt, G.A. (2004). Relapse prevention for alcohol and drug problems: that was Zen, this is Tao. *American Psychologist* 59 (4): L224.

Wong, P.T. (2011). Positive psychology 2.0: Towards a balanced interactive model of the good life. *Canadian Psychology/Psychologie Canadienne* 52 (2): 69.

Yakovenko, I., Quigley, L., Hemmelgarn, B.R. et al. (2015). The efficacy of motivational interviewing for disordered gambling: systematic review and meta-analysis. *Addictive Behavior* 43: 72–82. https://doi.org/10.1016/j.addbeh.2014.12.011.

CHAPTER 3

Key Clinical Processes in Lifestyle Medicine

Introduction

As a new speciality, Lifestyle Medicine has emerged to provide solutions to effective prevention, treatment, and oftentimes, reversal of lifestyle-related diseases, using therapeutic lifestyle interventions as the first approach. In doing so, there are unique ways of consultation that are evolving and providing the much-needed tools in the proper management of patients. There is an emphasis on lifestyle-related factors in a patient's history and physical examination. There are also screening and diagnostic tests that are relevant to lifestyle-related diseases which should be captured in the consultation. It is especially important to have a clear understanding of the interpretation of laboratory results for various illnesses, e.g. diabetes, using evidence-based guidelines. The interplay of the core aspects of lifestyle practices on health and well-being must be understood and this knowledge should guide the clinical processes. Good working knowledge of the chronic care model is vital to ensuring that the patient gets optimal care in the Lifestyle Medicine Clinic. The multi-disciplinary team plays a crucial role in the management of patients attending the Lifestyle Medicine Clinic. As we face a pandemic of lifestyle-related diseases, lots more patients require therapeutic lifestyle therapeutic interventions and clinical processes must evolve to meet this rising need. With the fast-evolving field of evidence in favour of the critical role played by Group Consultations and Virtual Group Consultations

Lifestyle Medicine: Essential MCQs for Certification in Lifestyle Medicine, First Edition.
Ifeoma Monye, Adaeze Ifezulike, Karen Adamson and Fraser Birrell.
© 2022 John Wiley & Sons Ltd. Published 2022 by John Wiley & Sons Ltd.

(including Shared Medical Appointments) in lifestyle medicine: one key process for the successful management of lifestyle-related diseases.

This chapter tests candidates on the knowledge of key clinical processes, including useful tools required in setting up and running a lifestyle medicine clinic.

1. Which of the following best represents key validated components of lifestyle medicine vital signs?

  a. AUDIT-C, physical activity, BMI

  b. BMI, blood pressure, sleep

  c. Emotional well-being, sleep, tobacco use

  d. Stress, sleep, alcohol consumption

2. In calculating the daily total energy expenditure, which of the following is most accurate about calorie expenditure?

  a. Daily total energy expenditure = sum of all activities

  b. Physical activity = 15 to > 30% of total

  c. Resting energy expenditure = 20–35% of total

  d. Thermic activity (effect of food) energy expenditure = 50% of total

3. Which of the following is most likely to have the highest daily energy expenditure?

  a. Physical activity

  b. Resting activity

  c. Sleep activity

  d. Thermic activity (effect of food)

4. Which of the following is most likely to have the least daily energy expenditure?

  a. Physical activity

  b. Resting activity

  c. Sleep activity

  d. Thermic activity (effect of food)

5. In carrying out a physical activity vital sign check, which of the following is the best question to assess cardiovascular exercise?

  a. 'On average, how many days in a month do you engage in moderate to strenuous exercise?'

  b. 'On average, how many minutes per day do you engage in moderate to strenuous exercise?'

  c. 'On average, how many months in a year do you engage in moderate to strenuous exercise?'

  d. 'On average, how many weeks in a month do you engage in moderate to strenuous exercise?'

6. A 65-year-old male patient diagnosed with type 2 diabetes says he walks briskly once or twice a week for 30 minutes each time. Which of the following is your best advice for him now?

    a. 'You are doing too much for your age and you should slow down'

    b. 'You are inactive and should increase your activity level'

    c. 'You are insufficiently active and should increase your activity level'

    d. 'You are sufficiently active and should maintain this level of activity'

7. In nutritional assessment of a patient, which of the following is a component of Michael Greger's daily dozen checklist?

    a. Chicken

    b. Exercise

    c. Lean meat

    d. Sleep

8. A 22-year-old female university student visits the clinic with complaints of inability to concentrate and feeling stressed out. You conclude from your history taking that there is a lot of background academic and relationship stress. You decide to use the perceived stress scale assessment to evaluate her. Which of the following best represents a question from the questionnaire?

    a. Have you felt angered by things that happened that were within your control?

    b. Have you felt confident in handling other people's personal problems?

    c. Have you felt unable to control the important things in your partner's life?

    d. Have you been upset because of something that happened unexpectedly?

9. Which of the following is the most accurate statement concerning the perceived stress scale assessment questionnaire?

    a. It is a 4-item questionnaire

    b. It is a 6-item questionnaire

    c. It is a 9-item questionnaire

    d. It is a 10-item questionnaire

10. Which of the following is most likely to directly contribute to chronic disease?

    a. Consumption of alcohol

    b. Physical activity

    c. Poor dietary patterns

    d. Underconsumption of calories

11. Which of the following statements most accurately describes the interpretation of the perceived stress scale assessment questionnaire?

    a. For the negatively framed questions, the scoring is (4) = Never

b. For the positively framed questions, the scoring is (4) = Never

c. The higher the score, the less perceived stress one is under

d. The lower the score, the more perceived stress one is under

12. A 77-year-old man attends the clinic with complaints of poor sleep. You decide to do a mini sleep assessment. Which of the following is the most appropriate information you will like to know about his sleep pattern?

    a. Perceived sleep quantity

    b. Typical day-time hours of sleep

    c. Typical nap hours of sleep

    d. Typical weekend hours of sleep

13. In treating a patient with tobacco dependence during a clinic visit, which of the following is the most appropriate advice to give to the patient?

    a. The amount of tobacco smoked is not as important as the number of years of smoking

    b. The damage to passive smokers over the years is negligible

    c. The number of years is just as important as the amount of tobacco smoked

    d. The number of years of smoking is not as important as the amount of tobacco smoked

14. A 40-year-old woman attends the clinic with stress-related illness. You find out that she recently lost her job. She has tried to cope in all sorts of ways but now admits to taking more alcohol than usual. You perform an AUDIT-C screen and decide to schedule a monthly clinic follow-up visit subsequently. Which of the following is the most appropriate action?

    a. Screen her at every visit

    b. Screen her every three months

    c. Screen her once a year

    d. Screen her twice a year

15. You are carrying out an AUDIT-C screening test on a patient. Which of the following is the most appropriate question?

    a. How often do you have one or more drinks on one occasion?

    b. How often do you have six or more drinks on one occasion?

    c. How often do you have ten or more drinks on one occasion?

    d. How often do you have two or more drinks on one occasion?

16. Which of the following best describes the body mass index (BMI)?

    a. Extreme Obesity $> 35\,\text{kg/m}^2$

    b. Obesity Class 2 is 35.0–$39.9\,\text{kg/m}^2$

    c. Obesity Class 3 > 35 kg/m²

    d. Overweight is 23.0–29.9 kg/m²

17. In the Framingham risk assessment screening tool, which of the following is most descriptive of the features tested?

    a. Assessment indicates the individual's risk of developing diabetes in the next 10 years

    b. Assessment indicates the individual's risk of developing myocardial infarction in the next five years

    c. The results apply to adults 18 years and older without heart disease or diabetes

    d. The results underestimate the risk for those with diabetes

18. Which of the following statements most accurately refers to the interpretation of the high sensitivity C-reactive protein (hsCRP)?

    a. Is the same as the standard C-reactive protein

    b. Measures high levels of C-reactive protein

    c. Measures lower levels of C-reactive protein

    d. Predicts risk of different diseases that cause inflammation

19. Which of the following nutrients is most likely to be deficient in the population?

    a. Calcium

    b. Vitamin A

    c. Vitamin D

    d. Zinc

20. Which of the following is most likely to be a component of the Framingham risk score?

    a. HDL cholesterol

    b. LDL cholesterol

    c. Triglycerides

    d. Weight status

21. Which of the following most accurately states the waist to hip measurement standards for men and women?

    a. Normal waist circumference in men is less than or equal to 122 cm

    b. Normal waist circumference in women is less than or equal to 88 cm

    c. Normal waist/hip ratio in men is less than or equal to 1.9

    d. Normal waist/hip ratio in women is less than or equal to 0.9

22. In the classification of Overweight and Obesity, which of the following best shows the interpretation of BMI?

    a. BMI of $< 18.5 \, \text{kg/m}^2$ is desirable for optimal weight management

    b. BMI of $18.5{-}24.9 \, \text{kg/m}^2$ is borderline overweight

    c. BMI of $25.0{-}29.9 \, \text{kg/m}^2$ is overweight

    d. BMI of $30.0{-}34.9 \, \text{kg/m}^2$ is obesity class 2

23. In the Finnish Diabetes Association Type 2 Diabetes Risk assessment form, which of the following statements is most accurate?

    a. Age of under 45 years gets a score of 1

    b. Body mass index of lower than $25 \, \text{kg/m}^2$ has a score of 2

    c. Total score estimates the risk of developing diabetes within 10 years

    d. Waist circumference is measured below the navel

24. In considering the disease risk for Type 2 Diabetes, hypertension and CVD, which of the following is the most significant association between the waist circumference and disease risk?

    a. Men with waist circumference of > 35 inches (88 cm) are at extremely high risk

    b. Overweight men with waist circumference of < 35 inches (88 cm) are at increased risk

    c. Waist circumference is considered increased if the waist is > 30 inches in women

    d. Waist/hip ratio is more predictive of risk of coronary events than BMI

25. Which of the following situations is the most appropriate to consider for testing for Diabetes?

    a. All adults who are overweight and have no other risk factor

    b. High-risk race or ethnicity patients who are of normal weight

    c. All women over 40 years of age

    d. Adults who are overweight with history of physical inactivity

26. Regarding hypertension, which of the following statements is the best advice for a newly diagnosed patient?

    a. A small decrease in systolic pressure can substantially reduce illness burden

    b. Prehypertension is diagnosed by systolic 110–129 mmHg and diastolic 80–89 mmHg

    c. Stage 1 Hypertension is diagnosed by systolic 130–149 mmHg and diastolic 90–99 mmHg

    d. The prevalence of hypertension reduces with age

27. In performing a risk factor assessment in Type 2 Diabetes, which of the following considerations most closely agrees with current recommendations?

a. A normal screening result requires bi-annual blood tests

b. Patients who are found to have pre-diabetes do not require intensive lifestyle intervention

c. Patients who are found to have pre-diabetes require intensive lifestyle intervention

d. Testing for Type 2 Diabetes should begin in all adults without identifiable risk factors at age of 50

28. Which of the following best describes the outcomes seen with a team approach?

a. Compared to standard care, educational interventions by GPs alone produced more sustained reduction in weight of patients after a year

b. Compared to standard care, educational interventions by GPs did not produce any sustained reduction in weights of patients after a year

c. Patients lost more weight after a year if the care was provided by a Dietician alone

d. Patients lost more weight after a year if the care was provided by a Doctor–Dietician team

29. In the Ornish Spectrum Program, which of the following best describes team roles?

a. Administrative assistant: Biometric assessment

b. Chef/Food services: Recipe referral

c. Exercise physiologist: PAR-Q assessment

d. Registered nurse: Consistent source of social support through change

The case history below is for Questions 30–33.

A 58-year-old African female presents to you to register for her primary health care needs and the following were found:

• Medical history: Obese, tired all the time, low moods
• Surgical history: Ovarian cystectomy
• Family history: T2DM, HTN, Prostate cancer in father
• Social history: Quit smoking a month ago; was a pack-a-day smoker, unemployed, going through a divorce and currently separated, lives alone
• Previously told she had a raised BP but didn't return for a follow-up

30. Which of the following tests best measures the general levels of inflammation in her body?

a. Electrolytes and urea

b. Full blood count

c. High-sensitivity C-reactive protein

d. Standard C-reactive protein

31. Which of the following tests best indicates her risk for heart disease and stroke?

a. Erythrocyte sedimentation rate

b. High sensitivity C-reactive protein

c. Sodium

d. Standard C-reactive protein

32. Her BP in the office measures 144/82 mmHg. Her BMI is 38 kg/m². Which of the following is the best next step in management?

a. Ambulatory home blood pressure monitoring

b. Lifestyle modification programme enrolment

c. Referral to the cardiologist

d. Start BP-lowering medications

33. You recommend that she needs to lose weight. You begin to discuss regular physical activity. She says she does not want to exercise as she doesn't feel any motivation to exercise. Which of the following is the next best step?

a. Discuss health risks in general

b. Refer her to a community gym

c. Refer her to a dance group

d. Refer her to a health coach

34. Which of the following most accurately represents research findings about a team approach in the clinical setting for lifestyle medicine?

a. Acceptance and referral to health programme were not dependent on the level of facilitation provided by physicians

b. Continuation and coordination of care were highly dependent on the patient's ability to pay for care

c. Importance of practice nurse's involvement in sustaining implementation of lifestyle changes was negligible

d. Lack of referral services for people at risk of developing cardiovascular disease threatens maintenance of lifestyle changes

35. In a lifestyle medicine clinic, office systems are best set up to do which of the following?

a. Effectively identify the patient's needs

b. Offer financial help where indicated

c. Offer high-tech laboratory tests

d. Remove troublesome patients from the registry

36. Which chronic care model feature best represents an acceptable model of care?

a. Group visits are superior to individual visits in optimization of lifestyle modification

b. Group visits are not designed to support lifestyle modification

c. Planned visits can optimize office visits to support lifestyle modification

d. There is no benefit for proactively prompting follow-up in lifestyle modification programmes

37. Which of these makes group visits the preferred choice when compared to individual visits?

a. Increased access and choice for patients

b. Increased waiting times for appointments

c. Increased patient satisfaction more than staff satisfaction

d. Increased staff satisfaction more than patient satisfaction

38. In the assessment of alcohol misuse, which of the following best describes the acronym 'AUDIT-C'?

a. Alcohol use and drugs in therapy consumption

b. Alcohol use disorders identification test consumption

c. Alcohol use diagnosis in therapy consumption

d. Alcohol use and disease identification test consumption

39. In administering the AUDIT-C questionnaire, which of these statements most accurately demonstrates the scoring system?

a. A total of at least 7 must be recorded for a positive test

b. A total of 0–6 represents low risk

c. A total of 5–7 indicates increasing risk

d. A total of 8–10 indicates possible dependence

40. Which of these questions best represents one of the three short AUDIT-C questions?

a. How many units of drink do you drink in a typical month when you are drinking?

b. How many units of drink do you drink in a typical week when you are drinking?

c. How many units of drink do you drink on a typical night out when you are drinking?

d. How many units of drink do you drink on a typical day when you are drinking?

41. A 60-year-old male patient attends the clinic with a new diagnosis of type 2 diabetes. The history reveals that he consumes a fair amount of alcohol. Which of the following is most likely to represent more units of alcohol when consumed?

a. A 440 ml can of 'super-strength' lager

b. A 75 cl bottle of wine (12%)

c. A pint of 'strong' or 'premium' beer, lager, or cider

d. Two pints of 'regular' beer, lager, or cider

42. In administering the AUDIT-C short-form questionnaire to a 60-year-old male patient with a new diagnosis of type 2 diabetes, which of the following best describes the score at which you go ahead to complete the remaining alcohol harm questions in order to obtain a full AUDIT-C score?

a. Score of 4 or more

b. Score of 5 or more

c. Score of 7 or more

d. Score of 10 or more

43. A 45-year-old male Afro-Caribbean patient attended the clinic with a blood pressure of 125/85 mmHg. He has a family history of hypertension. You counsel him about the importance of regular blood pressure checkups. Which of the following is the most appropriate advice at this time?

a. Screen for hypertension every day

b. Screen for hypertension every month

c. Screen for hypertension every six months

d. Screen for hypertension every two weeks

44. Small reductions in blood pressure (BP) have been found to reduce mortality from stroke and coronary heart disease. Which of the following best describes the % reduction in mortality from stroke?

a. A reduction in BP of 5 mmHg can result in 2% reduction in mortality from stroke

b. A reduction in BP of 5 mmHg can result in 5% reduction in mortality from stroke

c. A reduction in BP of 5 mmHg can result in 6% reduction in mortality from stroke

d. A reduction in BP of 5 mmHg can result in 14% reduction in mortality from stroke

45. Fasting lipids is a screening test relevant to lifestyle-related diseases. Which of the following statements most accurately describes interpretation of this test?

a. Elevations in triglycerides are often associated with high HDL

b. Particle size has been shown to help stratify risk

c. Particle density alone describes the function of cholesterol fractions

d. Raised LDL is preferable to raised HDL levels

46. Which of the following sets of investigations will be your best first choice in screening for a lifestyle-related disease?

a. Fasting lipids, hsCRP, HBA1C, vitamin D, selenium

b. Full blood count, fasting lipids, hsCRP, HBA1C, insulin

c. HOMA-IR, C-peptide, HBA1C, full blood count, zinc

d. Thyroid-stimulating hormone, T4, full blood count, HBA1C, chromium

47. Which of the following best describes the type of patient to screen for Type 2 Diabetes?

    a. Obese adult of Caucasian descent

    b. Obese woman who delivered a baby weighing 3.6 kg (8 pounds)

    c. Obese adult who is physically inactive

    d. Obese adult with a diabetic second-degree relative

48. In setting up a lifestyle medicine practice, a registry of patients should be in place, stratified by which of the following?

    a. Risk level based on the absence of healthy lifestyle practices

    b. Risk level based on the absence of lifestyle-related diseases

    c. Risk level based on the presence of healthy lifestyle practices

    d. Risk level based on the presence of lifestyle-related diseases

49. Which of the following best interprets the acronym 'PDSA', describing the process for health care service quality improvement?

    a. Plan, Deliver, Specify, Adopt

    b. Plan, Do, Study, Act

    c. Prepare, Demonstrate, Subject, Adapt

    d. Prepare, Diversify, Study, Approve

50. In the six-year initiative of the 'Prescription for Health' study by the Robert Wood Johnson Foundation (RWJF) and Agency for Healthcare Research and Quality (AHRQ), which of these best describes the four health risk behaviours that were targeted?

    a. Lack of physical activity, inadequate sleep, risky alcohol use, tobacco use

    b. Lack of physical activity, risky alcohol use, unhealthy diet, tobacco use

    c. Lack of physical activity, poor stress management, tobacco use, unhealthy diet

    d. Lack of physical activity, social isolation, risky alcohol use, tobacco use

51. In the 'Prescription for Health' study, which of the following is the most accurate finding?

    a. Primary care offices' capability and willingness to address health behaviour change in patients were not covered in this study

    b. Primary care offices were capable and willing to address health behaviour change in patients

    c. Primary care offices were capable but reluctant to address health behaviour in patients

    d. Primary care offices were neither capable nor willing to address health behaviour change in patients

52. In developing the chronic care model, which of these statements best fits the key processes to be considered?

    a. Encourage open, systematic handling of errors and issues of quality assurance

    b. Emphasize the physician's central role in the health care of the patients

    c. Installation of an electronic health record is mandatory in the coordination of care

    d. Self-management has not been shown to reduce symptoms and complications

53. Innovative Care for Chronic Conditions (ICCC) is a report by the World Health Organization that explains how health care systems can and must update their practices to care for chronic disease at each societal level. Which of the following best defines various levels of care?

    a. Macro level – health care organization and community

    b. Meso level – patient and family

    c. Meso level – health care organization and community

    d. Micro level – policy

54. Which of the following team roles has been most suitably matched?

    a. Chef/Food Services – recipe referral

    b. Exercise Physiologist – introduction to various mind–body techniques

    c. Registered Dietician – training in food selection and preparation

    d. Registered Nurse – biometrics assessment

55. Which of the following is best matched for the diagnosis of pre-diabetes?

    a. Fasting serum glucose equal to or less than 110 mg (6.1 mmol/l)

    b. HbA1C of 4.2–6.7% (31–49 mmol/l)

    c. Random serum glucose of more than or equal to 100 mg/l (5.6 mmol/l) but less than 126 mgl/L (7 mmol/l)

    d. Two-hour serum glucose in the 75 g OGTT of 140–199 mg/dl (7.8–11.0 mmol/l)

56. Which of the following best accounts for why Virtual Group Consultations are a desirable method of meeting patients' needs during the COVID-19 pandemic?

    a. Billable at group rates with no change in cost

    b. Easier access for COVID-19 testing

    c. It is a means of reaching out to remote patients

    d. Requires only one health professional to make it work

57. Which of the following statements has been found to be the most accurate finding in studies regarding Group Consultations (e.g. Shared Medical Appointments) in the practice of Lifestyle Medicine?

    a. Difficulty with maintaining patient confidentiality

    b. Increased provider satisfaction

    c. High-need patients do not benefit

    d. Reduced patient satisfaction

58. Which one of these is most beneficial when using Group Consultations (e.g. Shared Medical Appointments)?

    a. Greater patient education and lower hospitalization rates

    b. Improved access to a multi-disciplinary team with higher hospitalization rates

    c. Improved access to a multi-disciplinary team and time-consuming

    d. No effect on quality and outcome but contains cost

59. Which of the following is best matched for fitness testing in the lifestyle medicine clinic?

    a. Sit and reach for cardiorespiratory fitness

    b. Sit-ups for cardiorespiratory fitness

    c. Squats for muscular endurance

    d. Step testing for muscular endurance

Answers

1. **A** There are unique vital signs required for prescribing lifestyle medicine interventions. As reported in the Journal of the American Medical Association 2010 article, these include diet, physical activity, sleep, stress, emotional well-being, tobacco use, alcohol consumption, and BMI. Of all these, only physical activity, BMI, and AUDIT-C are validated at this time (Lianov and Johnson 2010).

2. **B** Daily total energy expenditure is a combination of resting energy expenditure, physical activity expenditure and thermic energy expenditure (Kelly and Shull 2019, p. 67).

3. **B** Resting energy expenditure = 60–70% of total (Kelly and Shull 2019, p. 67).

4. **D** Thermic activity = 10% of total (Kelly and Shull 2019, p. 67).

5. **B** This is one of the two-item exercise vital signs.

6. **C** According to the World Health Organization, the physical activity recommendation for adults and the elderly is at least 150 minutes of moderate-intensity exercise per week, e.g. brisk walking. (Kelly and Shull 2019, p. 189, 193).

7. **B** It is important to assess the daily consumption of healthy foods by the patient. Michael Greger's daily dozen checklist is a useful tool to have in the consulting room or have as an app that can be used by patients from the comfort of their home (see Tips Box 3.1; Kelly and Shull 2019).

TIPS BOX 3.1 | Greger's Daily Dozen Checklist

- Beans
- Berries
- Other fruits
- Cruciferous
- Greens
- Other vegetables
- Flaxseeds
- Nuts
- Spices (e.g. turmeric)
- Whole grains
- Beverages
- Exercise

Source: Kelly and Shull (2019).

---

8. **D** Apart from option D, the other correct questions include:

   Have you felt confident in handling your personal problems?
   Have you felt angered by things that happened that were not within your control?
   Have you felt unable to control the important things in your life?
   Kelly and Shull 2019, p. 69)

9. **D** The perceived stress scale assessment questionnaire is a 10-item questionnaire.

10. **C** Poor dietary patterns have been shown to contribute to numerous chronic diseases such as diabetes, hypertension, Alzheimer's disease, arthritis, irritable bowel syndrome, coronary heart disease, dyslipidaemia, metabolic syndrome, certain cancers, etc.

    The prevalence of chronic disease all over the world is rising exponentially and not sustainable by most health care systems. Healthy dietary patterns are diets that are high in fruits, vegetables, whole grains, beans, berries, nuts, seeds, low and non-dairy and lean protein, low in saturated fat, trans fat, sodium, and added sugar (Neuhouser, 2020).

11. **B** Scoring of the 10-item perceived stress scale assessment is as follows:

    - For the positively framed questions, the scoring is: (4) Never, (3) Almost never, (2) Sometimes, (1) Fairly Often, (0) Often
    - For the negatively framed questions, this is reversed: (0) Never, (1) Almost never, (2) Sometimes, (3) Fairly often, (4) Very often
    - The higher the score, the more perceived stress one is under

    (Kelly and Shull 2019, p. 69)

12. **D** The mini sleep assessment asks about three things:

    - Typical weekday hours of sleep
    - Typical weekend hours of sleep
    - Perceived sleep quality

    (Kelly and Shull 2019, p. 69)

13. **C** Passive smokers can suffer lung damage over years of being around a smoker. The number of cigarettes smoked is as important as the number of years smoked.

14. **A** As long as the patient is drinking alcohol regularly, screen her at every visit.

15. **B** See Tips Box 3.2

16. **B** See Tips Box 3.3

17. **D** The assessment indicates the patient's risk of myocardial infarction in the next 10 years. The assessment considers cholesterol, HDL-C, smoking, blood pressure, and medication for hypertension. The results underestimate the risk for those with diabetes. Results apply to adults 20 years and older without heart disease or diabetes.

18. **C** The high-sensitivity C-reactive protein test is a blood test that measures the lower levels of C-reactive protein. The protein measures general levels of inflammation in the body. It can be used to find the risk for heart disease and stroke in people who don't already have heart disease.

TIPS BOX 3.2 | Alcohol Use Disorders Identification Test Consumption (Audit-C)

AUDIT-C

Please circle the answer that is correct for you.

---

1. **How often do you have a drink containing alcohol?**   SCORE

| Never (0) | Monthly or less (1) | Two to four times a month (2) | Two to three times a week (3) | Four or more times a week (4) | _____ |

2. **How many drinks containing alcohol do you have on a typical day when you are drinking?**

| 1 or 2 (0) | 3 or 4 (1) | 5 or 6 (2) | 7 to 9 (3) | 10 or more (4) | _____ |

3. **How often do you have six or more drinks on one occasion?**

| Never (0) | Less than monthly (1) | Monthly (2) | Two to three times a week (3) | Four or more times a week (4) | _____ |

TOTAL SCORE

Add the number for each question to get your total score.   _____

Maximum score is 12. A score of ≥ 4 identifies 86% of men who report drinking above recommended levels or meet criteria for alcohol use disorders. A score of > 2 identifies 84% of women who report hazardous drinking or alcohol use disorders.

---

19. **D** Shortfall nutrients in the population include Vitamins A, D, E, C, calcium, iron (especially for women of menstruating age), magnesium, choline, potassium, and fibre. There is generally low consumption of these nutrients.

20. **A** The Framingham risk score is a gender-specific tool that helps in the assessment of risk level of coronary artery disease (CAD) over 10 years. The following are the components: age, gender, total cholesterol (TC), high-density lipoprotein (HDL), smoking habits, and systolic blood pressure.

21. **B** Waist circumference in men is less than 102 cm (< 40 inches), in women, it is 88 cm, waist /hip ratio in men is less than or equal to 0.9 and in women, it is less than or equal to 0.85.

22. **C** See Tips Box 3.3

TIPS BOX 3.3 | The Body Mass Index (BMI)

$BMI = \{Weight\ (lbs)/Height\ (in)^2\} \times 703$

OR

$BMI = Weight\ (kg)/Height\ (m)^2$

Classification BMI score (kg/m^2)

Underweight < 18.5

Normal 18.5–24.9

Overweight 25–29.9

Class 1 obesity 30.0–34.9

Class 2 obesity 35.0–39.9

Class 3 obesity BMI ≥ 40.0

---

23. **C** In the Type 2 diabetes risk assessment of the Finnish Diabetic Association, the waist circumference is measured at the level of the navel. Family history of type 1 and type 2 diabetes are components. Body mass index of lower than $25\,kg/m^2$ has a score of 1, while age of under 45 years gets a score of 0 (Kelly and Shull 2019).

24. **D** Screening for risk factors is important for prevention, diagnosis, and early treatment. As useful as the BMI is, the waist/hip ratio has been found to be more predictive of the risk for cardiovascular disease (Kelly and Shull 2019, p. 71).

25. **D** The following conditions warrant testing for diabetes; physical inactivity, a first-degree relative who has type 2 diabetes, hypertension, or patients on medication for hypertension, prediabetes, insulin resistance, polycystic ovary syndrome, high-risk race (Asian, Black, Latino, Native American, Pacific Islander) with overweight, gestational diabetes, history of cardiovascular disease (Kelly and Shull 2019, p. 71).

26. **A** Please see Tips Box 3.4: Classification of blood pressure in adults

27. **C** If there are no risk factors, the consensus is to begin screening for diabetes at age 45 and repeat every three years (Kelly and Shull, 2019, p. 74).

28. **D** Dietician care produced sustained weight loss, so did doctor's care but combined care by both produced more weight loss in patients (Flodgren et al. 2010).

29. **C** Biometric assessment is done by the exercise physiologist or physiotherapist. Recipe referral is done by the nutritionist. The health coach is the source of consistent social support throughout change (Ornish Spectrum Program 2020; http://deanornish.com/ornish-lifestyle-medicine/).

<table>
<tr><td colspan="3">TIPS BOX 3.4 | Joint National Committee, JNC 7 Classification of Blood Pressure in Adults</td></tr>
</table>

Blood pressure (BP) classification	Systolic BP (mmHg)	Diastolic BP (mmHg)
Normal	< 120	< 80
Prehypertension	120–139	80–89
Stage 1 Hypertension	140–159	90–99
Stage 2 Hypertension	> 160	> 100

30. C The most common way to measure inflammation is to check the CRP (hs-CRP). The high-sensitivity CRP is a blood test that measures lower levels of C-reactive protein. It measures the general levels of inflammation in the body and can be used to estimate the risk for heart disease and stroke in people who do not already have the disease.

31. B Hs-CRP can be used to estimate the risk for heart disease and stroke in people who don't already have the disease.

32. A Her BP shows a one-time office measurement of slightly raised systolic BP. So, ambulatory measurement is indicated to find out the actual value.

33. A She is at the precontemplation stage of the Prochaska and DiClemente's Cycle of change. All that is indicated at this stage is a general discussion of the health risks (Rippe 2019, p. 782).

34. D In the team approach of the management of lifestyle-related diseases, every team member provides a significant contribution to the care of the patient. Continuation of care is not dependent on the patient's ability to pay but on availability of different health care specialists and the level of coordination of care between various members of the multi-disciplinary team.

35. A Lifestyle medicine clinics should be set up to effectively identify the patient's needs. Heart sink patients should be accommodated and patients with financial needs should be sign-posted to appropriate agencies. Laboratory tests do not need to be high-tech; in fact, the opposite is the case.

36. C Group visits are not consistently superior to individual visits even though they have many benefits. They are designed to support lifestyle modification. It is highly beneficial to plan follow-up visits when patients are on a lifestyle medicine modification programme.

37. A Group Consultations, Group Visits, and Shared Medical Appointments are all alternative terms for the same underlying concept. They increase patient and staff satisfaction, increase access to health care services, and reduce waiting times (Birrell et al. 2020).

38. B See Tips Box 3.2: Scoring AUDIT-C

39. C See Tips Box 3.2: Scoring AUDIT-C

40. D See Tips Box 3.2: Scoring AUDIT-C

41. B 75cl bottle of wine (12%) is 9 units of alcohol. 440mls of super strength lager contains 4.5 units, One pint of strong beer is 3 units, Two pints of regular beer is 4 units..

42. B If you have a score of 5 or more with the short AUDIT-C form, you should go ahead to complete the remaining alcohol harm questions.

43. C Checking the BP every 6–12 months, when there is a positive family history, is recommended (Kelly and Shull 2019, p. 72).

44. D Small reductions in blood pressure can substantially reduce illness burden. As little as 2mmHg reduction in blood pressure can result in 6% reduction in mortality from stroke, and 4% reduction in mortality from coronary heart disease (Whelton 2002; Alexander et al. 2021; Kelly and Shull 2019, p. 73).

45. B Triglyceride elevations are often associated with low HDL and increased waist circumference. Particle size has been shown to help stratify risk; particle density alone does not completely account for the function of cholesterol fractions (Kontush and Chapman 2006).

46. B The lifestyle medicine investigations aim to check for a set of tests that provide further insight into the diagnosis or risk stratification of lifestyle-related diseases, whose root cause is usually underlying chronic systemic inflammation.

47. C The best fit here is the inactive obese adult. At-risk races include Asian, Black, Latin Americans, Native Americans, and Pacific Islanders.

48. A Patients being registered in a lifestyle medicine practice should be stratified in such a way as to find out early on the lifestyle practices that may put them at risk of developing any of the lifestyle-related diseases.

49. B PDSA stands for Plan, Do, Study, and Act. When setting up a new service, it is useful to set up systems to ensure the service runs smoothly. Looking to achieve small-scale improvements over short periods of time will usually require several cycles of PDSA to create the desired change. Persistence and review of services with regular evaluation is key.

50. B See Prescription for health: http://www.prescriptionforhealth.org/. Accessed 20 November 2020.

51. B See Prescription for health

52. A Open, systematic handling of errors, in a non-judgemental manner and issues of quality assurance are to be encouraged. The patient has a significant role to play in the health care. Self-management has been shown to reduce symptoms and complications and installation of electronic health records (EHR) is not mandatory.

53. C See the WHO document on innovative care for chronic conditions: Building Blocks for Action (WHO 2002).

54. D The recipe referral is done by the nutritionist, training in food selection and preparation by the chef, and introduction to mind-body techniques by the stress management specialist. See Ornish Spectrum Program. Available here: http://deanornish.com/ornish-lifestyle-medicine/

55. D Prediabetic lab tests should be done on a fasting sample to obtain a more accurate interpretation.

56. C There are numerous benefits of Virtual Group consultations, including improved access to care, benefits to patients as well as benefits to the health care team (Birrell et al. 2020).

57. B Confidentiality is maintained during Group Consultations. All participants sign the confidentiality form. High-need patients benefit from this method of consultation and there is increased patient satisfaction (Eisenstat et al. 2012; Egger et al. 2014).

58. A There is improved access to a multi-disciplinary team with lower hospitalization rates, less waiting time and reduced costs (Trento et al. 2002).

59. C Cardiorespiratory fitness: step testing

Muscular endurance: squats, push-ups, sit-ups
Flexibility: sit and reach
Body composition: skin callipers
(Kelly and Shull 2019, p. 73)

References

Alcohol Unit Reference. https://alcoholchange.org.uk/alcohol-facts/interactive-tools/unit-calculator

Alexander, R.M., Madhur, M.S., Harrison, D.G., et al., Hypertension Clinical Presentation. https://emedicine.medscape.com/article/241381-clinical. Last accessed on 23 June 2021

Birrell, F., Lawson, R., Sumego, M. et al. (2020). Virtual group consultations offer continuity of care globally during Covid-19. *Lifestyle Medicine*. https://doi.org/10.1002/lim2.17.

Egger, G. et al. (2014). Shared medical appointments – an adjunct for chronic disease management in Australia? *Australian Family Physician* 43 (3): 151–154.

Eisenstat, S.L.S., Carlson, K., and Ulman, K. (2012). *Putting Group Visits into Practice: a Practical Overview to Preparation, Implementation, and Maintenance of Group Visits at Massachusetts General Hospital*. Massachusetts General Hospital.

Flodgren, G. et al. (2010). Interventions to change the behaviour of health professionals and the organisation of care to promote weight reduction in overweight and obese adults. *Cochrane Database of Systematic Reviews* (3).

Kelly J, Shull J. The Lifestyle Medicine Board Review Manual. 2019 American college of Lifestyle Medicine

Kontush, A. and Chapman, M.J. (2006). Functionality defective high-density lipoprotein: a new therapeutic target at the crossroads of dyslipidaemia, inflammation and atherosclerosis. *Pharmacological Reviews* 58 (3): 342–374.

Lianov, L. and Johnson, M. (2012). Physician competencies for prescribing lifestyle medicine. *JAMA* 304(2):202-203. https://doi.org/10.1001/jama.2010.903. PMID: 20628134.

Neuhouser, M.L. (2020). Red and processed meat: more with less? *American Journal of Clinical Nutrition* 111 (2): 252–255.

Ornish Spectrum Program (2020). http://deanornish.com/ornish-lifestyle-medicine/ (accessed 22 November 2020).

Prescription for Health (2020). http://www.prescriptionforhealth.org/ (accessed 25 November 2020).

Rippe, J.M. (2019). Lifestyle Medicine. 3rd Edition. CRC Press Taylor and Francis Group: USA.

Trento, M. et al. (2002). Lifestyle intervention by group care prevents deterioration of Type 2 diabetes: a 4-year randomised controlled clinical trial. *Diabetologia* 45 (9): 1231–1239.

Whelton, P.K. (2002). Primary Prevention of hypertension: clinical and public health advisory from The National High Blood Pressure Education Program. *JAMA* 288 (15): 1882–1888.

WHO (2002). Building Blocks for Action. https://www.who.int/chp/knowledge/publications/icccreport/en/q (accessed 20 November 2020).

CHAPTER 4

Physician Health

Introduction

Why should we pay attention to a physician's health? Do a physician's healthy lifestyle practices make a difference in the clinical care of his patients? Physicians are people and patients too (although there is evidence, they are not the best or even good patients), so the choices they make as individuals can have direct and indirect effects on their health. One of the strongest predictors of health promotion during routine consultations is whether the physician practices a healthy lifestyle. Key aspects are whether dietary and exercise choices physicians make have any bearing on their views and ability to effect behaviour change for patients. But health advocacy is also a valuable tool whereby lifestyle physicians can leverage their impact on a community. So, an understanding of this is valuable. As is realizing medical students are already developing their own distinct lifestyle behaviours, which is likely to profoundly impact both their own future behaviour as doctors and their potential impact on patients. This chapter tests the candidates on barriers to physicians' health and how the health of physicians can affect their patients' health.

1. Which of the following would be the most important for physicians to consider when developing an action plan for their own health?

   a. Allergies and food intolerance

   b. Barriers to change, strategies, and actions to overcome identified barriers

   c. Limitations and social support

   d. Referral to an appropriate specialist

Lifestyle Medicine: Essential MCQs for Certification in Lifestyle Medicine, First Edition.
Ifeoma Monye, Adaeze Ifezulike, Karen Adamson and Fraser Birrell.
© 2022 John Wiley & Sons Ltd. Published 2022 by John Wiley & Sons Ltd.

2. A physician was drawing up his own action plan. Which of the following is least likely to be a feature of his goals?

   a. Sensitive

   b. Measurable

   c. Achievable

   d. Relevant

3. Which of the following best describes some of the features of the acronym SMART in goal setting?

   a. Measurable, Relevant, and Time-bound

   b. Relevant, Actionable, and Sensible

   c. Sensitive, Relevant, and Time-bound

   d. Specific, Manageable, and Relevant

4. A review of 24 studies of Physicians' Physical Activity (PA) habits (Lobelo and de Quevedo 2016) showed that:

   a. Physically active physicians are more likely to provide PA counselling to their patients

   b. There was no significant positive association between physicians' PA habits and counselling frequency

   c. Physical activity habits and counselling frequency were inversely associated

   d. Physically active physicians are less likely to provide PA counselling to their patients

5. Which option best summarizes why physicians make poor patients?

   a. Inevitable dichotomy between doctor and patient roles

   b. Multifactorial, including work pressure, personality traits, less likely to seek care

   c. Structural risk factors not amenable to change

   d. They are healthy and do not generally get ill

6. Which of the following best describes Health Advocacy by physicians?

   a. It does not usually require liaising with community organizations and/or other partners

   b. It involves identifying wellness needs of a community

   c. It is a solo effort

   d. It is not a co-ordinated effort to promote a public health issue

7. Which best describes health advocacy?

   a. Always includes information on enacting change

   b. Always requires the advocate to be an agent of change

   c. Can include information on enacting change or involve being an agent of change

   d. Never involves the advocate being an agent of change

8. Which of these best describes Lifestyle Medicine core competency 2?

   a. Physicians should seek to practise healthy behaviour only at work

   b. Physicians should create home environments that support healthy behaviour

   c. Physicians should practise healthy behaviours and create school, work, and home environments that support healthy behaviours

   d. Physicians should work with the health care teams to promote healthy meals in the workplace

9. Which of these best describes physicians' advocacy?

   a. Doctors make poor health advocates in the community

   b. Extending impact of clinical work to the community is not feasible

   c. The clinical encounter provides an opportunity for the physician to advocate healthy behaviour to the patient

   d. The skills used in the clinic cannot be extended to community advocacy

10. Which of the following best describes the advantages of physician involvement in community health advocacy?

    a. Better health outcomes only if services are doctor-led

    b. More credibility for achieving the health goal

    c. Poorer engagement

    d. Poorer health-seeking behaviour

11. When considering how doctors can be involved in community advocacy, which of the following is the least likely?

    a. Be a health resource for the community

    b. Health talks with the media

    c. Offer expertise to elected community officials

    d. Provide advice on an individual basis

12. In a study of 498 primary care physicians by Bleich et al. (2012), which of the following best describes the percentage who were overweight or obese?

    a. 10–20%

    b. 30–40%

    c. 50–60%

    d. 80–90%

13. In 2013, Holtz surveyed Canadian medical students. Which of the following percentages best describes the proportion who reported levels of exercise that did not meet Canadian Society for Exercise Physiology Guidelines?

    a. 10%

    b. 40%

    c. 80%

    d. 90%

14. Bazargan et al. (2009) surveyed nearly 800 California physicians. Which of the following best represents the percentage who never or occasionally ate breakfast?

   a. 7%

   b. 17%

   c. 27%

   d. 37%

15. Bazargan et al. (2009) surveyed nearly 800 California physicians in 2009. Which of the following best describes the areas in which they are poor role models?

   a. Clinical skills, empathy, and exercise

   b. Sleep, clinical skills, and working > 60 h/wk

   c. Sleep, clinical skills, and empathy

   d. Sleep, exercise, and working > 60 h/wk

16. Which of the following best describes the findings of Bleich et al. (2012) in 'Impact of Physician BMI on Obesity Care and Beliefs'?

   a. Physicians in the normal BMI category were less likely to believe that physicians should model healthy weight-related behaviours

   b. Results suggest that less normal weight physicians provided recommended obesity care to their patients and felt confident doing so

   c. A higher percentage of normal BMI physicians believed that overweight/obese patients would be less likely to trust weight loss advice from overweight/obese doctors

   d. Physicians with a higher BMI had greater confidence in their ability to provide diet and exercise counselling

17. Which of the following best describes the findings in the study on exercise behaviour and attitudes among fourth-year medical students at the University of British Columbia (Holtz et al. 2013)?

   a. 6% of students met the Canadian Society for Exercise Physiology 2011 recommendations for PA.

   b. Students who engaged in more strenuous PA were more likely to perceive exercise counselling as being highly relevant to future clinical practice

   c. 26% thought that their training in Exercise Counselling was less than extensive

   d. Attitudes towards healthy living were not related to PA levels

18. Bazargan et al. (2009) surveyed nearly 800 California physicians. Which of the following was most likely to be associated with the physicians' excessive number of work hours?

   a. Eating breakfast

   b. Lack of exercise

   c. Lower levels of stress

   d. Sleeping an average of seven hours per night

19. Which of the following best describes the findings of Bleich et al. (2012) in 'Impact of Physician BMI on Obesity Care and Beliefs'?

    a. Physicians with normal BMI were more likely to engage their obese patients in weight loss discussions as compared to overweight/obese physicians

    b. Physicians with high BMI were more likely to engage their obese patients in weight loss discussions as compared to normal weight physicians

    c. Physicians with low BMI were more likely to engage their obese patients in weight loss discussions as compared to overweight/obese physicians

    d. Overweight physicians were less likely to engage obese patients in weight loss discussions as compared to normal BMI physicians.

20. Impact of Physician BMI on Obesity Care and Beliefs (Bleich et al. 2012) showed that:

    a. Physicians with high BMI had greater confidence in their ability to provide diet and exercise counselling to their obese patients compared to normal BMI physicians

    b. Physicians with low BMI had greater confidence in their ability to provide diet and exercise counselling to their obese patients compared to overweight/obese physicians

    c. Physicians with low or high BMI had greater confidence in their ability to provide diet and exercise counselling to their obese patients compared to normal BMI physicians

    d. Physicians with normal BMI had greater confidence in their ability to provide diet and exercise counselling to their obese patients compared to overweight/obese physicians

21. Impact of Physician BMI on Obesity Care and Beliefs (Bleich et al. 2012) revealed that:

    a. A higher percentage of low BMI physicians believed that overweight/obese patients would be less likely to trust weight loss advice from overweight/obese doctors

    b. A higher percentage of normal BMI physicians believed that overweight/obese patients would be less likely to trust weight loss advice from overweight/obese doctors

    c. A higher percentage of high BMI physicians believed that overweight/obese patients would be less likely to trust weight loss advice from overweight/obese doctors

    d. The same percentage of low, high, and normal BMI physicians believed that overweight/obese patients would be less likely to trust weight loss advice from overweight/obese doctors

22. In 2013, Helfand and Mukamal published their paper 'Do healthcare workers practise what they preach?' Which of the following do they say health care workers more likely to report doing?

    a. Have a personal physician

    b. Admit to recent heavy or binge drinking

    c. Have a recent dental check-up

    d. Wear a seat belt

23. Do healthcare workers practise what they preach? Helfand and Mukamal 2013 revealed that there were significant differences between healthcare workers (HCWs) and non-HCWs in which of the following areas:

    a. Recent smear (Papanicolaou) test

    b. Being overweight or obese

    c. Drinking and driving

    d. Binge drinking or heavy drinking

24. In 2014, Lobelo et al. published 'The Evidence in Support of Physicians and Health Care Providers as Physical Activity Role Models'. Which of the following best describes their findings?

    a. A negative association between HCPs' Physical Activity habits and counselling frequency

    b. That physically active physicians and other HCPs are more likely to provide PA counselling to their patients

    c. Physicians cannot become powerful PA role models

    d. Inactive HCPs are more likely to provide credible PA counselling

25. Oberg and Frank (2013) studied the relationship between physician's health practices and patient's health practices. Which of the following describes their findings least well?

    a. Addressing providers' own health behaviours is key to substantially increasing health-promotion counselling in general practice.

    b. Physician counselling is strongly unrelated to one's own health practices

    c. Physicians can positively influence patients' health habits by counselling them about prevention and health-promoting behaviours

    d. Providers benefit from interventions that help them adopt healthier lifestyles – this benefit is not only for their personal health, but for the health of their entire patient population, which is likely to profit from more efficient and effective health promotion counselling

Answers

1. **B** While the other options would apply to some physicians, most are affected by barriers to change, including overwork, shift patterns, dietary and exercise habits. For example, like many workers, physicians often feel they have no time to exercise, but data from the UK Biobank shows a strong protective effect from 'active commuting', especially cycling to work (Celis-Morales et al. 2017).

2. **A** SMART objectives are Specific, Measurable, Achievable, Relevant and Time-bound.

3. **A** Revision! See above.

4. **A** Lobelo and de Quevedo (2016) reported 'Most (19 out of 24) analytic studies reported a significant positive association between HCPs' PA habits and counselling frequency, with odds ratios ranging between 1.4 and 5.7 ($P < 0.05$), in six studies allowing direct comparison. This review found consistent evidence supporting the notion that physically active physicians and other HCPs are more likely to provide PA counselling to their patients and can indeed become powerful PA role models.'

5. **B** This is not a simple issue, with multiple factors involved. While there is a dichotomy, this is not inevitable and is amenable to change. For example, the practitioner support programme achieves health professional outcomes better than usual, not worse. (Wessely and Gerada 2013).

6. **C** Health advocacy refers to activities related to ensuring access to care, navigating the system, mobilizing resources, addressing health inequities, influencing health policy, and creating system change (Hubinette et al. 2017; see Tips Box 4.1).

7. **B** 'Always' and 'never' are rarely the best option in Lifestyle and other variants of Medicine. Oandasan (2005) did a qualitative community study which showed there were two types of health advocates: (i) informants – providing information to those who can enact change, or (ii) change agents – initiating, mobilizing, and organizing ways to systematically modify policies or procedures that negatively affect patients/communities.

8. **C** Core competencies were published in 2010 (Lianov and Johnson 2010) and include a comprehensive list of suggested competencies (see Tips Boxes 1.2 and 4.2), although arguably group consultations might justify inclusion when these are revised, as a key driver behaviour change and personalized patient-centred care.

9. **C** Although health advocacy includes the community, of the options presented, the clinical encounter is the best description.

10. **B** While advocacy can involve other team members, credibility rather than uniquely better outcomes is a key advantage.

11. **D** Note the contrast from Q. 9: Compared to these options, individual advice does not map as well to health advocacy.

TIPS BOX 4.1 | Health Advocacy Practice Points

- To be competent health advocates, physicians must understand the factors that create health inequities and recognize how they impact the lives of their patients
- Although it is clear that efforts to improve health of an individual or population must consider 'upstream' factors, how this is operationalized in medicine and medical education is controversial
- Health advocacy is both a mindset and a multifaceted set of skills that includes ensuring access to care, navigating the health care system, mobilizing resources, addressing health inequities, influencing health policy, and creating system change
- Numerous curricular interventions have been described but successful integration of health advocacy into medical programs will require a broader examination of processes, practices, and values throughout medicine and medical education and will involve education enterprises, organizations, and institutions as well as the communities they serve
- There is both an essential cognitive foundation and experiential/workplace learning component to teaching and learning health advocacy
- The UBC Health Advocacy Framework suggests different types, levels, and approaches to advocacy resulting in four quadrants of advocacy activities (shared/directed agency/activism)

Source: Hubinette et al. (2017).

TIPS BOX 4.2 | Updated Lifestyle Medicine Competencies 2020

A. Leadership
  1) Promote healthy behaviours to prevent, treat, and reverse disease
  2) Develop leadership culture and environments supporting, healthy behaviours

B. Knowledge
  3) Show knowing evidence on certain lifestyle changes improves patients' health outcomes
  4) Show knowledge of lifestyle medicine modalities to prevent, treat, and reverse disease
  5) Describe ways physicians engage with patients/families can improve health behaviours

C. *Assessment Skills*
  6) Assess bio-, psycho-, social and environmental behaviours and resulting health outcomes
  7) Assess readiness, willingness, and ability for health behavioural change

D. *Service Delivery*
  8) Perform lifestyle-specific history and physical examination, including lifestyle "vital signs"
  9) Do and interpret apt tests to screen, diagnose, treat and monitor chronic diseases
  10) & 11) Use recognized guidelines to help patients self-manage lifestyles/ treat disease
  12) & 15) Establish effective therapeutic relationships effecting and sustaining behaviour change with evidence-based counselling methods, tools and follow-up.
  13) Help patients/families with evidence-based, SMART action plans/lifestyle prescriptions
  14) Refer patients to appropriate healthcare professionals for lifestyle-related conditions

E. *Therapeutic Alliance*
  16) Identify meaningful health behaviour changes consistent with their vision and values
  17) Manage health behaviour change with empathy and support

F. *Use of Office and Community Support*
  18) Use an interdisciplinary healthcare team and support a team approach
  19) Apply office routines supporting lifestyle medical care e.g. decision support/ referral
  20) Support quality improvement for lifestyle interventions with process/ outcome data
  21) Use apt community referral resources to support implementation, including apps

Adapted from *Lianov et al, 2020*

12. **C** This was a study of 500 physicians, excluding two who were underweight ($BMI < 18.5\,kg/m^2$). The majority were male (67%), white (70%), age 40 or older (72%), overweight or obese (53%), and general internists (55%; Bleich et al. 2012).

13. **B** In this survey of 883 medical students, where 546 (62%) responded. 64% of responders met the Canadian Society for Exercise Physiology, 2011 recommendations for PA (Holtz et al. 2013).

14. **C** While many of the health behaviours in this anonymous survey (Bazargan et al. 2009) were unequivocally negative: 13% reported using sedatives/tranquillizers, 4% self-reported recent marijuana use, > 6% screened positive for alcohol abuse, 5% for gambling problems; and 35% reported 'no'/'occasional' exercise. Eating breakfast or not was less obviously

negative behaviour: 27% self-reported 'never' or 'occasionally' eating breakfast. There is a lack of evidence that eating breakfast is a healthy behaviour, despite many attempts to demonstrate this (Moberly 2019).

15. D 34% reported ≤ 6h of sleep daily, while 21% self-reported working > 60 h/wk (Bazargan et al. 2009).

16. C While unsurprising, the knowledge that role-modelling for obesity in this setting is also effective is empowering for both physicians and patients.

17. B Similarly, role-modelling for physical activity also operated in the antici-pated (and hoped for) direction.

18. B Available time and healthy living ethos would both predict lack of exer-cise as the key variable associated with excessive hours of work (Bazargan et al. 2009). It is noteworthy that eating breakfast was not associated with these healthy behaviours.

19. A This is a variation on the theme: Q. 16 is about beliefs and this is about actions. This can be rationalized that normal BMI physicians are on firmer ground- both in raising and role-modelling this issue.

20. D Another variation about confidence, which can differ from competence, beliefs, and actions – again the normal BMI physicians are confident and empowered in this area.

21. B A final variation about beliefs, on the theme of those in glass houses being less likely to throw stones.

22. A Of these options, only having a personal physician was more common in health care workers. Smoking, HIV risk behaviours, sunburn, and being dissatisfied with life were equivalent.

23. D Health care workers were less likely to report binge drinking (RR 0.88, 95%CI 0.79–0.98) or heavy drinking (RR 0.76, 95% CI 0.66–0.88) than others, with no significant differences in the other health behaviours.

24. B The main comparison shown was with physicians' physical activity and PA counselling frequency with the recommendation that the quality of counselling is included in future studies.

25. B There is a strong relationship between physician counselling and health practices. So, this is the least suitable option.

References

Bazargan, M., Makar, M., Bazargan-Hejazi, S. et al. (2009). Preventive, lifestyle, and personal health behaviors among physicians. *Academic Psychiatry* 33 (4): 289–295.

Bleich, S.N., Bennett, W.L., Gudzune, K.A., and Cooper, L.A. (2012). Impact of physician BMI on obesity care and beliefs. *Obesity* 20 (5): 999–1005. https://doi.org/10.1038/oby.2011.402.

Celis-Morales, C.A., Lyall Donald, M., Welsh, P. et al. (2017). Association between active commuting and incident cardiovascular disease, cancer, and mortality: prospective cohort study. *BMJ* 357: j1456.

Helfand, B.K. and Mukamal, K.J. (2013). Healthcare and lifestyle practices of healthcare workers: do healthcare workers practice what they preach? *JAMA Internal Medicine* 173 (3): 242–244. https://doi.org/10.1001/2013.jamainternmed.1039. PMID: 23247811.

Holtz, K.A., Kokotilo, K.J., Fitzgerald, B.E., and Frank, E. (2013). Exercise behaviour and attitudes among fourth-year medical students at the University of British Columbia. *Canadian Family Physician* 59 (1): e26–e32.

Hubinette, M., Dobson, S., Scott, I., and Sherbino, J. (2017 Feb). Health advocacy. *Medical Teacher* 39 (2): 128–135. https://doi.org/10.1080/0142159X.2017.1245853.

Lianov L, Adamson K, Kelly J, Matthews S, Palma M, Rea B. Lifestyle Medicine Competencies. Revised Version. Lifestyle Medicine Global Alliance: November 2020.

Lianov, L. and Johnson, M. (2010). Physician competencies for prescribing lifestyle medicine. *JAMA* 304 (2): 202–203. https://doi.org/10.1001/jama.2010.903. PMID: 20628134.

Lobelo, F. and de Quevedo, I.G. (2016 Jan). The evidence in support of physicians and health care providers as physical activity role models. *American Journal of Lifestyle Medicine* 10 (1): 36–52. https://doi.org/10.1177/1559827613520120. Epub 2014 Jan 21. PMID: 26213523; PMCID: PMC4511730.

Moberly, T. (2019). Unscrambling the evidence for breakfast. *BMJ* 364: l456.

Oandasan, I.F. (2005). Health advocacy: bringing clarity to educators through the voices of Physician Health Advocates. *Academic Medicine* 80 (10): S38–S41.

Oberg, E. and Frank, E. (2013). Physicians' health practices are better than patients'. *JAMA Internal Medicine* 173 (12): 1155–1156. https://doi.org/10.1001/jamainternmed.2013.6512. PMID: 23797167.

Wessely, A. and Gerada, C. (2013). When doctors need treatment: an anthropological approach to why doctors make bad patients. *BMJ* 347: f6644.

CHAPTER 5

Nutrition Science, Assessment and Prescription

Introduction

Nutrition science has evolved with the growing understanding of the relationship between nutrient consumption, actions, interactions, and balance in relation to health and disease. There is therefore a need for a rigorous, science-based approach to nutrition. This chapter covers the science of nutrition, including biochemistry, anthropomorphic and nutritional assessment, food labels, calorific density, fat, cholesterol, and mineral intake. Management options include weight management, dietary advice, behaviour change and holistic approaches, including the core competencies in Lifestyle Medicine. Through the examples shared we are trying to foster an understanding that there is no single dietary intervention that has yet shown superiority in robust trials, so our approach needs to be flexible, mapped to the individual and evidence-based, rather than dogmatic and relying on any single philosophy. However, there are many pieces of evidence supporting a wholly or predominantly plant-based diet, the adoption of which also supports planetary medicine and sustainability goals. We provide some questions to test candidates' understanding of assessing and prescribing nutrition, interpreting food labels and the different approaches to weight management.

Lifestyle Medicine: Essential MCQs for Certification in Lifestyle Medicine, First Edition.
Ifeoma Monye, Adaeze Ifezulike, Karen Adamson and Fraser Birrell.
© 2022 John Wiley & Sons Ltd. Published 2022 by John Wiley & Sons Ltd.

1. When assessing a patient for the first time, a basic nutrition assessment should be undertaken. Which of the following best describes a basic nutrition assessment?

a. It always requires follow-up by a registered dietician

b. It can be performed by a Lifestyle Medicine Physician

c. It requires an in-depth laboratory assessment

d. Referral to a Registered Dietician is required in the first instance

2. When performing an anthropometric assessment, which of the following is most accurate?

a. Body Mass Index (BMI) accounts for muscle/bone mass

b. BMI correlates accurately across all ethnic groups

c. The equipment can be calibrated every three to four years

d. Percentage body fat is a more accurate assessment of nutritional status than BMI

3. When performing a primary biochemical assessment, which of the following combinations would be most appropriate?

a. Potassium, Glucose, Calcium

b. Sodium, Haematocrit, HbA1c

c. Sodium, Potassium, Calcium

d. Sodium, Potassium, Ferritin

4. Which of the following best describes a key component of the practice of Lifestyle Medicine?

a. Emphasis on diagnostic laboratory tests

b. Emphasis on vitamin supplements

c. Pharmaceuticals as first line of treatment

d. Use of whole food plant-based nutrition

5. Which of the following most closely describes best practice in Lifestyle Medicine?

a. Emotional wellness plays a minimal role

b. Nutrition must follow a named diet to yield lasting results

c. Medication remains the mainstay of management

d. Sleep prescription is an important pillar in management of many chronic diseases

6. Which of the following best applies to weight management?

a. Eating quickly can aid weight loss

b. Eating slowly can hinder weight loss

c. Keeping a food diary can aid weight loss

d. Physical activity is more important than calorie restriction

7. A basic nutrition assessment is a key part of the initial assessment. Which of the following are key elements?

    a. Biochemical data from laboratory tests are not required

    b. Encompasses cultural beliefs

    c. Must be performed by a Lifestyle Medicine Physician

    d. Weight, height, and basal metabolic rate

8. Which of the following most appropriately describes a Lifestyle Medicine setting?

    a. Inpatient surgical care centre

    b. Primary, secondary, or tertiary care clinics that incorporate group consultations in the management of their patients

    c. Super-specialist diagnostic centre

    d. Tertiary care consultant-delivered service

9. A patient is keen to understand more about food labelling. Which of the following best describes the categories used in food labelling?

    a. Food containing 1 g/100 g of Fat is Amber

    b. Food containing 3–20 g/100 g of Fat is Amber

    c. Food containing 10–18 g/100 g of Fat is Green

    d. Food containing > 20 g/100 g of Fat is Amber

10. During a Lifestyle Medicine consultation, a patient asked about calorific density of foods. Which of the following has the highest calorific density?

    a. Confectionary

    b. Fruits

    c. Mushrooms

    d. Nuts

11. Which of the following has the highest calorific density?

    a. Bread

    b. Grain-based desserts

    c. Pizza

    d. Sweetened beverages

12. A 50-year-old was found to have high cholesterol. She asks about the cholesterol content of foods. Which of the following has the highest cholesterol content?

    a. Beef

    b. Dairy

    c. Eggs

    d. Processed meat

13. During a Lifestyle Medicine consultation, the concept of saturated and unsaturated fats was discussed. Which of these has the least saturated fat content?

    a. Chicken

    b. Dairy

    c. Herbs and spices

    d. Nuts

14. A 60-year-old man with hypertension was advised to reduce his salt intake. Which of the following has the highest sodium content?

    a. Bread

    b. Cold cuts

    c. Pizza

    d. Processed meat

15. Concerning trans fat, which of these contains the least?

    a. French fries

    b. Grain-based processed foods

    c. Margarine

    d. Potato chips

16. In the therapeutic approaches used in Lifestyle Medicine, which of these therapeutic interventions has been most appropriately represented?

    a. Cognitive Behavioural Therapy is seldom used

    b. Group consultations have been found to be effective

    c. Lifestyle Medicine approaches have not been found to be effective in management of communicable diseases

    d. Motivational counselling is more effective than medications in severe depression

17. Which of the following is the best food source of magnesium?

    a. Fish

    b. Herbs and spices

    c. Legumes

    d. Seeds

18. Comparing Lifestyle Medicine and Preventive Medicine, which of these best compares their approaches?

    a. Lifestyle Medicine practice is the same as Preventive Medicine in approach

    b. Medication is the 'end' in both fields of Medicine

c. Personalized care is a key feature in both fields of Medicine

d. Preventive Medicine, unlike Lifestyle Medicine, emphasizes population-based interventions

19. Which of the following is a key process in health coaching for behavioural change in Lifestyle Medicine?

a. Assessing client's readiness for change

b. Changing the lifestyle of a client

c. Enforcing behavioural change in the client

d. Setting goals for the client

20. In a city in the USA, there are 5000 dwellers. Using the national average, what is the most likely estimate of those with diabetes?

a. 10

b. 279

c. 465

d. 956

21. Which of the following is the most appropriate behaviour change technique for the behaviour change process?

a. In the early stages, use cognitive behavioural therapy

b. In the later stages, use motivational interviewing

c. In all stages, use motivational interviewing

d. In all stages, use positive psychology

22. When considering intensive medication intervention in the management of Type 2 Diabetes Mellitus, which of the following is most accurate?

a. Always aim for the lowest possible glucose level

b. Increased insulin dosing is associated with a reduction in the risk of cardiovascular heart disease

c. Increased insulin dosing is associated with an increased risk of cancer

d. The intensive arm of the ACCORD trial was continued because it showed much promise in glucose control

23. Which of the following best reflects the physician competencies for prescribing Lifestyle Medicine?

a. Physician engagement with the patient has not been shown to improve patient outcome

b. Physicians' role model and practise healthy personal behaviours

c. The healthcare provider should avoid engagement with the patient

d. The physician helps patients sustain healthy lifestyle practices with no need to refer to other specialities

24. When considering Type 2 Diabetes and lifestyle, which of the following statements is the most accurate?

a. Around 50% of the increase in Type 2 Diabetes Mellitus in the second half of the twentieth century is linked to lifestyle

b. Around 50% of those with pre-diabetes will develop Type 2 Diabetes Mellitus within five years

c. Diabetes is not preventable by lifestyle intervention alone

d. For children born after 2000, 33% of men and 38% of women will develop Diabetes

25. In Physician Competencies in Lifestyle Medicine, which of the following best explains the important processes involved in the assessment of a patient?

a. Assessment of social, psychological, and biological predispositions and the desired health outcome is very important

b. Assessment of environmental factors is the most important aspect

c. Assessment of family readiness and willingness is more important than client's readiness and willingness

d. Assessment of employer's readiness and willingness is more important than family readiness and willingness

26. Health coaching in Lifestyle Medicine is more likely to succeed in which of the following situations?

a. Readiness of the patient and members of their support group to make a health behaviour change

b. Readiness of the patient and their community to make a health behaviour change

c. Readiness of the patient and their employer to make health behaviour change

d. Readiness of the patient and their family to make health behaviour change

27. A 53-year-old lady with a recent diagnosis of ischaemic heart disease asked about the development of atherosclerosis. Which of the following are risk factors for the development of atherosclerosis?

a. Being inactive

b. Being overweight

c. Dyslipidaemia

d. Hypotension

28. His BMI is 40. He has dyslipidaemia, severe left hip pain and is keen to have Lifestyle Medicine interventions for his condition. For the past five years, his treatment consists of Atorvastatin, Metformin, and Soluble Insulin. Based on current evidence, which of the following will be the most effective option of therapeutic Lifestyle intervention treatment for him now?

    a. Intensive therapeutic lifestyle change treatment

    b. Non-intensive therapeutic lifestyle change treatment

    c. Intensive therapeutic lifestyle change treatment followed by therapeutic lifestyle change

    d. Non-intensive therapeutic lifestyle change treatment followed by therapeutic lifestyle change

29. Which of the following statements is the most accurate when considering a plant-based diet?

    a. It typically lowers HDL cholesterol

    b. It typically lowers LDL cholesterol

    c. It typically lowers triglycerides

    d. No difference in cholesterol is seen when compared with other diets

30. In the scientific foundation of the Healthy Doctor-Healthy Patient project (Frank et al. 2013), which of the following most accurately represents the findings in this study?

    a. Counselling patients makes a difference in patients' habits and in their health

    b. North American physicians tend to live just as long as their peers

    c. Physicians live longer than their contemporaries because they have access to better medical care

    d. Physicians with poor health habits are more likely to advise their patients about preventive habits

31. In a 2001 study by Jenkins et al., looking at a diet high in fibre from fruits and vegetables, which of the following statements is the most accurate?

    a. Cholesterol reduction by a plant-based diet was found to be equivalent to a therapeutic statin dose

    b. Faecal bile acid output remained the same

    c. Maximum lipid reductions occurred within one month

    d. The study lasted for three months

32. In the 1998 Lifestyle Heart trial by Ornish et al., the experimental group patients demonstrated a reduction in reported frequency of angina after one year. Which of the following is the most accurate estimate of the reduction seen?

    a. 10%

    b. 50%

c. 60%

d. 90%

33. When considering the results of the 2012 low-carbohydrate/high-protein diet and incidence of cardiovascular diseases in Swedish women study, which of the following statements is the most accurate?

a. A low-carbohydrate, high-protein diet, used on a regular basis and without consideration of the nature of carbohydrates or the source of protein is associated with decreased risk of CVD

b. A one-tenth decrease in carbohydrate intake or increase in protein intake were all statistically significantly associated with increasing incidence of cardiovascular disease overall

c. The participants consisted of teenaged girls and women

d. There is a reduction in incidence of cardiovascular disease with low-carbohydrate, high-protein diet

34. A study in 2009 by Barnard et al. compared the treatment of Type 2 Diabetes Mellitus with a low-fat vegan diet versus a conventional diabetes diet. Which of the following statements best describes their findings?

a. Both diets were associated with sustained reductions in weight and plasma lipid concentrations.

b. Neither diet showed significant reduction in weight or plasma lipid concentrations

c. The low-fat vegan diet was associated with reduction in weight and plasma lipid concentration while the diabetic diet was associated with only weight loss

d. Weight loss was significantly different between the two groups

35. When considering fats, which of the following statements is the most accurate?

a. Harmful saturated fats should be eaten in moderate amounts

b. Trans fats should be completely eliminated

c. Trans fat foods should be minimized

d. Trans fats should be generously prescribed

36. Which of the following is best described as harmful saturated fat?

a. Lauric acid

b. Myristic acid

c. Palmitic acid

d. Stearic acid

37. Which of the following typically contains the most lauric acid?

a. Butter

b. Cashews

    c. Egg yolks

    d. Salmon

38. When considering dark chocolate, which of the following statements is the most accurate?

    a. Associated with lower LDL Cholesterol compared to other saturated fats

    b. Does not contain stearic acid

    c. Contains saturated fatty acid that is more likely to convert to cholesterol esters

    d. Associated with lower HDL

39. Which of the following statements is most accurate with regard to palmitic acid?

    a. Increased consumption has not been shown to lead to increased heart disease

    b. It is the most common type of saturated fat

    c. It can be safely consumed in moderate amounts

    d. More found in butter than in palm oil

40. Which of the following is likely to be the best source of fibre?

    a. Green vegetable

    b. Legumes

    c. Oatmeal

    d. Wheat-containing cereal

41. Which of the following cooking methods is most likely to reduce advanced glycation end-products?

    a. Boiling

    b. Frying

    c. Grilling

    d. Smoking

42. Which of the following cancers is most likely to be associated with a poor intake of fruits and vegetables?

    a. Breast

    b. Ovarian

    c. Pancreatic

    d. Prostate

43. Geoff, a 46-year-old man, has been advised to increase his fibre intake by his GP to help with bowel function. Which of the following best describes the amount of fibre per day he should ideally aim for?

    a. 15 g

    b. 25 g

c. 20 g

d. 35 g

44. Susan consults you as she has been advised to reduce the amount of sugary drinks she gives to her obese children. She tells you that she finds the food labels confusing. She notes that her son's favourite drink contains 25 g of added sugar/100 ml. She wants to know how many spoonfuls of sugar that means. Which of the following is the best approximation of the sugar content?

a. 4 teaspoons

b. 6 teaspoons

c. 8 teaspoons

d. 10 teaspoons

45. Linda, a 51-year-old lady, has been advised to increase her intake of calcium. She wants to know what amount of calcium she should aim to take daily. Which of the following best describes the amount an adult woman should take daily?

a. 200 mg

b. 300 mg

c. 1000 mg

d. 1600 mg

46. Stephen is 52 years old and recently diagnosed with hypertension. You advise him to reduce salt intake and he wants to know how much salt he is to take daily. Which of the following best describes the maximum daily amount of salt for adults?

a. 3 g

b. 6 g

c. 10 g

d. 16 g

47. Which of the following is the most likely strategy to be used in successful weight loss programs?

a. Bi-monthly weighing

b. Increasing screen time

c. Monthly weighing

d. Setting SMART goals

48. Roger is 50 years old and has elevated total cholesterol. He wishes to reduce the fat content of his diet. Which of the following is the best approximation of the percentage of total energy requirements from fat?

a. 5–10%

b. 10–15%

c. 15–20%

d. 25–30%

49. Sharon is 28 years old and has just had a positive pregnancy test. She currently drinks eight strong coffees a day. Which of the following represents the best approximation of the total amount of caffeine she should consume daily in pregnancy?

    a. 100 mg

    b. 200 mg

    c. 300 mg

    d. 400 mg

50. Which of the following best describes the reduction in LDL cholesterol seen with the portfolio diet?

    a. 8%

    b. 18%

    c. 28%

    d. 38%

51. Which of the following interventions utilized a comprehensive lifestyle intervention and showed significant regression in coronary artery stenosis at 12 months?

    a. Lyon Diet Heart Study

    b. Mediterranean diet

    c. Ornish diet

    d. Portfolio diet

52. Pierce et al. (2007) conducted a study in obese women with breast cancer. They looked at the effect of physical activity and fruit and vegetable intake on breast cancer survival. Which of the following best describes their findings?

    a. Diet and not physical activity impacted positively on survival

    b. Physical activity and not diet impacted positively on survival

    c. When corrected for fruit and vegetable intake and physical activity, obese women had a higher mortality than non-obese women

    d. When corrected for fruit and vegetable intake and physical activity, obese women had a similar mortality to non-obese women

53. The Diabetes Prevention Program (DPP) trial showed that lifestyle intervention reduced progression to diabetes from impaired glucose tolerance. Which of the following best describes the reduction seen?

    a. 38%

    b. 48%

    c. 58%

    d. 68%

54. In the Diabetes Prevention Program (DPP) trial, metformin reduced the development of diabetes. Which of the following best describes the reduction seen?

a. 21%

b. 31%

c. 41%

d. 51%

55. Which of the following foods is least likely to increase inflammatory markers?

a. Blackberries

b. Bread

c. Butter

d. Pork

56. A patient asked why dark chocolate is often described as more beneficial than milk chocolate. Which of the following is the most accurate?

a. It contains saturated fatty acid that is more likely to convert to cholesterol esters

b. It does not contain stearic acid

c. It is associated with a lower HDL level

d. It is associated with a lower LDL cholesterol compared to other saturated fats

57. A 2010 study by Keranis et al. showed a reduction in COPD mortality with a diet high in anti-oxidant foods. Which of the following best describes the risk reduction seen?

a. 4%

b. 14%

c. 24%

d. 34%

58. A 2010 study by Keranis et al. showed a reduction in COPD mortality with a diet high in antioxidant foods. Which of the following best describes the lung function findings seen?

a. A decrease in FEV1

b. A decrease in FVC

c. An increase in FEV1

d. No change in FVC

59. Which of the following best describes the findings of Lin et al. in their 2010 study on diet and kidney function?

a. Higher animal fat intake increased the risk of microalbuminuria

b. Higher beta carotene intake increased the risk of eGFR decline

c. Higher fructose intake increased the risk of microalbuminuria

d. Higher vegetable fat intake increased the risk of microalbuminuria

60. Chiba et al. (2010) compared a semi-vegetarian diet to usual treatment of patients with Crohn's disease. Which of the following best describes their findings?

a. A semi-vegetarian diet reduced the risk of relapse

b. A semi-vegetarian diet increased the risk of relapse

c. Optimal medication led to less relapse than a semi-vegetarian diet

d. No difference was seen in the risk of relapse

61. In 2012, a study in Swedish women looked at the impact of a low-carbohydrate, high-protein diet and the incidence of cardiovascular diseases. Which of the following best describes the findings?

a. A low-carbohydrate, high-protein diet used on a regular basis and without consideration of the nature of carbohydrates or the source of protein associated with decreased risk of CVD

b. A one-tenth decrease in carbohydrate intake or increase in protein intake were all statistically significantly associated with increasing incidence of cardiovascular disease overall

c. A reduction in the incidence of cardiovascular disease was seen with a low-carbohydrate, high-protein diet

d. The participants consisted of teenaged girls and women

62. A study in 2009 by Barnard et al. compared the treatment of people with Type 2 Diabetes Mellitus with a low-fat vegan diet versus a conventional diet. Which of the following best describes the findings?

a. Both diets were associated with sustained reductions in weight and plasma lipid concentrations

b. Neither diets showed significant reduction in weight or plasma lipid concentrations

c. The low-fat vegan diet was associated with reduction in weight and plasma lipid concentration while the diabetic diet was associated with only weight loss

d. Weight loss was significantly different between the two groups

63. Which of these statements best explains research findings of the impact of improving diet on chronic illnesses?

a. Dietary improvement has negligible impact on cataracts

b. Dietary improvement often results in a flare of inflammatory bowel disease

c. Dietary measures have a positive association with the incidence of asthma

d. Dietary measures impact positively on chronic obstructive airway disease

64. Which of these statements best explains the findings of a predominantly plant-based diet on health?

a. A protein-based diet is positively associated with increased risk of many cancers as well as Type 2 Diabetes Mellitus

b. Eating a plant-based diet has been found to cut the risk of some cancers

c. Plant-based nutrition delays gastric emptying and increases incidence of bowel cancers

d. There is currently insufficient evidence to support shifting food intake to a more plant-based diet to optimize health

65. Which of the following best outlines the impact of dietary berries on glycemic and cardiovascular parameters in Type 2 Diabetes Mellitus?

a. Berries are best consumed as part of a healthy and balanced diet

b. Berries have negligible effect on blood pressure, glycaemic, and lipid profiles

c. Cranberries and blueberries contribute to hyperinsulinemia in overweight or obese adults with insulin resistance

d. Raspberries and strawberries worsen postprandial hyperglycaemia and promote metabolic syndrome

66. Which of the following best describes the findings of Dietary Intake of total, animal, and vegetable protein and risk of Type 2 Diabetes Mellitus in the European Prospective Investigation into Cancer and Nutrition (EPIC) study?

a. All protein types increased risk of diabetes

b. All protein types were found to have a negligible effect on diabetes

c. Animal protein was associated with increased risk of diabetes

d. Vegetable protein was associated with increased risk of diabetes

67. Which of the following is the most appropriate finding from the updated nurses' study of the impact of eggs on diabetics?

a. Diabetics who ate more than one egg a week doubled their risk of cardiovascular disease

b. Eating lots of eggs had a negligible effect on the risk of Diabetes Mellitus and on glycaemic control

c. Eating lots of eggs improved the health and glycaemic control of diabetics

d. No overall association between moderate egg consumption and risk of Type 2 Diabetes Mellitus

68. Which of these statements is the best concerning the effect of fibre on glycaemic control?

a. Fibre intake improved glycaemic control by production of short-chain fatty acids

b. Fibre intake is positively associated with worsened glycaemic control

c. Fibre intake was found to be a risk factor for bowel cancer in diabetics

d. Fibre intake worsens glycaemic intake by slowing down absorption, thereby increasing blood sugar

69. Which of these statements is the most appropriate concerning plant-based nutrition and effect on the disease?

a. Plant-based nutrition is a major factor in causing mortality from constipation

b. Plant-based nutrition is associated positively with the incidence of hypertension

c. Plant-based nutrition has been found to normalize angiogenesis, thus reducing co-morbid disease

d. Plant-based nutrition results in reduced gastric motility leading to increased blood sugar absorption

Answers

1. **B** A basic nutrition assessment can be undertaken by anyone with the relevant skills

2. **D** Gallagher et al. highlight the importance of body fat measurement, especially as an individual ages, where BMI can remain constant but body fat percent increases (Gallagher et al. 2000).

3. **B** This combination will allow the assessment of the presence of diabetes and hydration level as a good primary assessment.

4. **D** A predominantly plant-based, whole food diet is one of the pillars of Lifestyle Medicine.

5. **D** Deprescribing is an important concept in Lifestyle Medicine, not medication. Sleep is key.

6. **C** Eating slowly can aid weight loss and keeping a food diary is important for the individual to understand what exactly they are eating. Whilst physical activity is important, calorie restriction is more important for weight loss (Hollis et al. 2008).

7. **B** An awareness of all the elements that influence an individual's eating habits is important when performing a nutrition assessment (Peterson and Maryniuk 1996).

8. **B** LM can be undertaken in any health care environment as long as the practitioner has the appropriate skills.

9. **B** Food labels use a traffic light system to aid interpretation for content with red being high, amber medium, and green low. https://www.nutrition. org.uk/healthyliving/helpingyoueatwell/324-labels.html?start=3

10. **A** Sweets and confectionary are very calorie-dense.

11. **B** Grain-based deserts have the highest calorie density.

12. **C** The average egg contains 177 mg of cholesterol.

13. **A** Chicken is lean meat. Hence, it has the lowest saturated fat content.

14. **C** As a rule, processed foods have higher sodium content.

15. **D** Potato chips (crisps) have the least trans fats of the foods stated.

16. **B** Group consultations have a unique potential for delivering system-wide benefits through a patient-centred approach (Jones et al. 2019). https:// bslm.org.uk/lifestyle-medicine/group-consultations/

17. **D** Seeds are an excellent source of magnesium.

18. **D** Lifestyle Medicine can be defined as the systematic practice of assisting individuals and families to adopt and sustain behaviours that can improve health and quality of life, whilst preventive medicine is population-based (Clarke and Hauser 2016).

19. A   Key features of effective health coaching include goal setting, motivational interviewing, and collaboration with health care providers (Palmer and Whybrow 2003; Olsen and Nesbitt 2010).

20. C   10.5% of the US population and 4% of the UK population have diabetes.

21. D   Positive psychology can build patient confidence, emphasize the patients' current skills and abilities, reinforce autonomy, and enhance resilience (Fredrickson 2001).

22. C   Insulin is a growth factor and stimulates cancer cell growth in vitro and, as such, hyperinsulinaemia is assumed to have a cancer-promoting effect (Vigneri et al. 2020).

23. D   The following are the physician competencies for prescribing Lifestyle Medicine (Lianov and Johnson 2010; See Tip Boxes 1.2 and 4.2):
Leadership
Promote healthy lifestyle behaviours
Practice healthy lifestyle behaviours
Knowledge
Demonstrate knowledge that lifestyle can positively affect health outcomes
Describe ways in which physicians can effect health behaviour change
Assessment skills
Assess social, psychological, and biologic predispositions
Assess readiness to change
Perform Lifestyle Medicine-focused history, physical and testing
Management skills
Use nationally recognized practice guidelines
Establish effective relationships with patients
Collaborate with patients and their families to develop specific action plans like Lifestyle Medicine prescriptions
Help patients manage and sustain healthy lifestyle practices including referrals as necessary
Office and community support
Have the ability to practise in interdisciplinary and community teams
Apply office systems and technologies to support Lifestyle Medicine
Measure processes and outcomes
Use appropriate community referral resources to support the implementation of healthy lifestyles

24. D   The data from CDC estimates published in 2003 are sobering with even higher rates estimated among Hispanics (Narayan et al. 2003).

25. A   See answer to Q. 23.

26. A   Readiness of the patient and their support group is key to success.

27. C   Newer risk factors, including impaired fasting glucose, triglycerides, and triglyceride-rich lipoprotein remnants, lipoprotein(a), homocysteine, and high-sensitivity C-reactive protein, contribute to an increased risk of coronary and cardiovascular diseases (Fruchart et al. 2004).

28. C This combination is most likely to achieve the step changes needed and potentially sustain them (Mechley and Dysinger 2015).

29. B A vegetarian diet was associated with lower mean concentrations of total cholesterol, low-density lipoprotein cholesterol, and high-density lipoprotein cholesterol compared with consumption of omnivorous diets (Yokoyama et al. 2017).

30. A In addition to counselling patients making an impact on their behaviours, there is a positive relation between physicians' and patients' preventive health practices (Frank et al. 2013).

31. A Individuals were fed a diet very high in fibre from fruits and vegetables. The levels fed were those which had originally inspired the dietary fibre hypothesis related to colon cancer and heart disease prevention and also may have been eaten early in human evolution.

Compared with the starch-based and low-fat diets, the high-fibre vegetable diet resulted in the largest reduction in low-density lipoprotein (LDL) cholesterol and the greatest faecal bile acid output, faecal bulk, and faecal short-chain fatty acid outputs (Jenkins et al. 2001).

32. D Comprehensive lifestyle changes were made and maintained for five years, leading to a reduction in angina frequency and a reduction in cardiac events (Ornish et al. 1998).

33. B Low-carbohydrate, high-protein diets, used on a regular basis and without consideration of the nature of carbohydrates or the source of proteins, are associated with increased risk of cardiovascular disease (Pagona et al. 2012).

34. A Both diets were associated with sustained reductions in weight and plasma lipid concentrations. In an analysis controlling for medication changes, the low-fat vegan diet appeared to improve glycaemia and plasma lipids more than did conventional diabetes diet recommendations (Barnard et al. 2009).

35. B Trans fats are formed through industrial processes. They increase LDL cholesterol and decrease HDL cholesterol (Mayo Clinic 2020).

36. C Palmitic acid is one of the commonest saturated fats. It is found in palm oil, butter, cheese, milk, and meat (NCBI 2020a).

37. A Lauric acid is found naturally in various plant and animal fats and oils, and is a major component of coconut oil and palm kernel oil (NCBI 2020b).

38. A Total cholesterol and LDL were reduced by eating dark chocolate (Lee et al. 2017).

39. B See answer to Question 36.

40. B The following are good sources of fibre (British Nutrition Foundation 2018):
- Wholegrain breakfast cereals, wholewheat pasta, wholegrain bread and oats, barley, and rye
- Fruits such as berries, pears, melons, and oranges
- Vegetables such as broccoli, carrots, and sweetcorn

- Peas, beans, and pulses
- Nuts and seeds
- Potatoes with skin

41. A   Dry heat promotes AGE formation whilst moist heat reduces it (Uribarri et al. 2010).

42. A   A very-low-fat, high-fibre diet combined with daily exercise results in major reductions in risk factors for breast cancer while subjects remained overweight/obese (Barnard et al. 2006).

43. D   Daily fibre recommendations are 25 g for women, ideally above 40 g a day, and 38 g for men, ideally above 45 g a day (Kelly and Shull 2019b).

44. B   One teaspoon contains 4.2 g of sugar.

45. C

Calcium: Recommended daily amount	
Men	
19–50 years	1000 mg
51–70 years	1000 mg
71 years and older Women	1200 mg
19–50 years	1000 mg
51 years and older	1200 mg

Calcium and Calcium Supplements (2020)

46. B   Adults should eat no more than 6 g of salt a day, which is around 1 teaspoon (Salt: the facts 2018).

47. D   Setting SMART goals is a useful strategy for any goal in Lifestyle Medicine.

48. D   Energy from total fats should be 25–30% of total diet energy, with a reduction in saturated fats to < 10% (Egger et al. 2017a).

49. C   A limit of 400 mg of caffeine daily is recommended for adults, reducing to 300 mg daily in pregnant women (Egger et al. 2017b).

50. C   The control, statin, and dietary portfolio groups had mean (SE) decreases in low-density lipoprotein cholesterol of 8% (2%) ($P = 0.002$), 31% (4%) ($P < 0.001$), and 29% (3%) ($P < 0.001$), respectively. Respective reductions in C-reactive protein were 10% (9%) ($P = 0.27$), 33% (8%) ($P = 0.002$), and 28% (11%) ($P = 0.02$). The significant reductions in the statin and dietary portfolio groups were all significantly different from changes in the control group. There were no significant differences in efficacy between the statin and dietary portfolio treatments (Jenkins et al. 2003).

51. C   Regression of coronary atherosclerosis was seen in the group adhering to intensive lifestyle changes (Ornish et al. 1998).

52. D   The study showed that breast cancer survivors who consume a healthy diet and are physically active may increase their years of survival after diagnosis. When corrected for fruit and vegetable intake and physical activity, obese women had a similar mortality to non-obese women (Pierce et al. 2007; Kelly and Shull 2019b, p. 171).

53. C   Lifestyle intervention resulted in a 58% reduction in the incidence rate of diabetes in the Diabetes Prevention Program (DPP – Diabetes Prevention Program Research Group 2002).

54. B   The incidence of diabetes was reduced by 58% with the lifestyle intervention and by 31% with metformin, as compared with placebo. These effects were similar in men and women and in all racial and ethnic groups (Diabetes Prevention Program Research Group 2002).

55. A   Blackberries and other berries are antioxidant-rich, whereas the other foods mentioned are pro-inflammatory (Kelly and Shull 2019a, p. 139).

56. D   Dark chocolate is associated with lower LDL cholesterol compared to other saturated fats. Other health benefits of dark chocolate include antioxidant, improvement in endothelial function, vascular function, insulin sensitivity and it is majorly beneficial in cardiovascular disease (Patel et al. 2019).

57. C   The study showed a protective effect of fruit against COPD. A 100 g increase in fruit intake was associated with a 24% lower COPD mortality risk (Keranis et al. 2010; Walda et al. 2002).

58. C   An increase in FEV1 was noted in the intervention group suggesting that a dietary shift to higher-antioxidant food intake may be associated with improvement in lung function (Keranis et al. 2010).

59. A   The study showed that higher dietary intake of animal fat and two or more servings per week of red meat may increase risk for microalbuminuria. Lower sodium and higher β-carotene intake appear protective (Lin et al. 2010).

60. A   Chiba et al investigated the use of a semi-vegetarian diet in 22 adult patients with Crohn's disease who were in remission over a two-year period. 73% achieved compliance, the remission rate was 100% at one year and 92% at two years.

61. D   Low-saturated fat dietary program has been found to delay progression in early-stage Multiple Sclerosis. Frequency of multiple sclerosis is inversely related to the amount of saturated animal fat consumed daily in various countries (Kadoch 2012).

62. C   A one-tenth decrease in carbohydrate intake or increase in protein intake were all statistically significantly associated with increasing incidence of cardiovascular disease overall. A low carbohydrate-high protein diet may be nutritionally acceptable if the protein is mainly of plant origin and the reduction of carbohydrates applies mainly to simple and refined ones (Lagiou et al. 2012).

63. D   Dietary improvements which include encouraging high intake of fruits, nuts and seeds, vegetables, fish, legumes, and limited intake of meat and dairy products have been shown to have favourable health outcomes with lower risk for chronic illnesses (Echouffo-Tcheugui and Ahima 2019).

64. B   There is convincing evidence that plant-based dietary intake (vegetable fats, dietary fibres, and phytonutrients such as phytosterols) has a beneficial effect on all aspects of health (Trautwein and McKay 2020).

65. A   Despite the beneficial effects of berries on diabetes prevention and management (such as ameliorating postprandial hyperglycaemia and hyperinsulinaemia in overweight or obese adults with insulin resistance, and in adults with the metabolic syndrome, they must be consumed as part of a healthy and balanced diet (Calvano et al. 2019).

66. C   Higher intake of total protein was associated with a lower risk of all-cause mortality, and intake of plant protein was associated with a lower risk of all-cause and cardiovascular disease mortality. Vegetable protein was not associated with an increased risk of diabetes (Kelly and Shull 2019a; Naghshi et al. 2020).

67. D   Results from this updated meta-analysis showed no overall association between moderate egg consumption and risk of Type 2 Diabetes Mellitus. The authors noted, however, significant differences by geographic region, for instance, each 1 egg/d was associated with higher Type 2 Diabetic risk among US studies but not among European studies (Drouin-Chartier et al. 2020).

68. A   A high-fibre, plant-based diet helps reverse diabetes and is associated with a lower risk of diabetes (Kelly and Shull 2019a).

69. C   Polyphenols derived from dietary plant intake have protective effects on vascular endothelial cells, possibly as antioxidants that prevent the oxidation of low-density lipoprotein (Tuso et al. 2015; Sanchez et al. 2019).

References

Barnard, N.D., Cohen, J., Jenkins, D.J. et al. (2009). A low-fat vegan diet and a conventional diabetes diet in the treatment of type 2 diabetes: a randomized, controlled, 74-wk clinical trial. *American Journal of Clinical Nutrition* 89 (5): 1588S–1596S.

Barnard, R.J., Gonzalez, J.H., Liva, M.E., and Ngo, T.H. (2006). Effects of a low-fat, high-fiber diet and exercise program on breast cancer risk factors in vivo and tumor cell growth and apoptosis in vitro. *Nutr Cancer* 55 (1): 28–34. https://doi.org/10.1207/s15327914nc5501_4;British Nutrition Foundation (2018). https://www.nutrition.org.uk/healthyliving/basics/fibre.html (accessed 31 December 2020). Calcium and calcium supplements (2020). https://www.mayoclinic.org/

healthy-lifestyle/nutrition-and-healthy-eating/in-depth/calcium-supplements/art-20047097 (accessed 31 December 2020).

Calvano, A., Izuora, K., Oh, E.C. et al. (2019). Dietary berries, insulin resistance and type 2 diabetes: an overview of human feeding trials. *Food & Function* 10 (10): 6227–6243.

Chiba, M., Abe, T., Tsuda, H. et al. (2010). Lifestyle-related disease in Crohn's disease: relapse prevention by a semi-vegetarian diet. *World Journal of Gastroenterology* 16 (20): 2484–2495. https://doi.org/10.3748/wjg.v16.i20.2484.

Clarke, C.A. and Hauser, M.E. (2016). Lifestyle medicine: a primary care perspective. *Journal of Graduate Medical Education* 8 (5): 665–667.

Diabetes Prevention Program Research Group (2002). Reduction in the incidence of type 2 diabetes with lifestyle intervention or metformin. *New England Journal of Medicine* 346 (6): 393–403.

Drouin-Chartier, J.P., Schwab, A.L., Chen, S. et al. (2020). Egg consumption and risk of type 2 diabetes: findings from 3 large US cohort studies of men and women and a systematic review and meta-analysis of prospective cohort studies. *The American Journal of Clinical Nutrition*.

Echouffo-Tcheugui, J.B. and Ahima, R.S. (2019). Does diet quality or nutrient quantity contribute more to health? *The Journal of Clinical Investigation* 129 (10): 3969–3970.

Egger, G.J., Binns, A.F., Rossner, S.R. et al. (2017a). Lifestyle Medicine, 3ee, 146. Australia: McGraw-Hill Education.

Egger, G.J., Binns, A.F., Rossner, S.R. et al. (2017b). Lifestyle Medicine, 3ee, 158. Australia: McGraw-Hill Education.

Frank, E., Dresner, Y., Shani, M., and Vinker, S. (2013). The association between physicians' and patients' preventive health practices. *CMAJ: Canadian Medical Association Journal = journal de l'Association medicale canadienne* 185 (8): 649–653. https://doi.org/10.1503/cmaj.121028.

Fredrickson, B.L. (2001). The role of positives emotions in positive psychology: the broaden-and-build theory of positive emotions. *The American Psychologist* 56 (3): 218–226.

Fruchart, J.-C., Nierman, M.C., Stroes, E.S.G. et al. (2004). New risk factors for atherosclerosis and patient risk assessment. *Circulation* 109 (suppl 1): III15–III19. https://doi.org/10.1161/01.CIR.0000131513.33892.5b. PMID: 15198961.

Gallagher, D., Heymsfield, S.B., Heo, M. et al. (2000). Healthy percentage body fat ranges: an approach for developing guidelines based on body mass index. *The American Journal of Clinical Nutrition* 72 (3): 694–701.

Hollis, J.F., Gullion, C.M., Stevens, V.J. et al. (2008). Weight loss during the intensive intervention phase of the weight-loss maintenance trial. *American Journal of Preventive Medicine* 35 (2): 118–126.

Jenkins, D.J., Kendall, C.W., Popovich, D.G. et al. (2001). Effect of a very-high-fiber vegetable, fruit, and nut diet on serum lipids and colonic function. *Metabolism.* 50 (4): 494–503.

Jenkins, D.J.A., Kendall, C.W.C., Marchie, A. et al. (2003). Effects of a dietary portfolio of cholesterol-lowering foods vs Lovastatin on serum lipids and C-reactive protein. *JAMA.* 290 (4): 502–510. https://doi.org/10.1001/jama.290.4.502.

Jones, T., Darzi, A., Egger, G. et al. (2019). Systems approach to Embedding Group Consultations in the NHS. *Future Healthcare Journal* 6: 8–16. https://doi.org/10.7861/futurehosp.6-1-8.

Kadoch, M.A. (2012). Is the treatment of multiple sclerosis headed in the wrong direction? *Canadian Journal of Neurological Sciences* 39 (3): 405–405.

Kelly, J. and Shull, J. (2019b). Lifestyle Medicine Board Review Manual, 2ee, 132. Section 5 Nutrition Science, Assessment and Prescription.

Kelly, J. and Shull, J. (2019a). Foundations of Lifestyle Medicine: Lifestyle Medicine Board Review Manual, 2ee, 115–181. American College of Lifestyle Medicine.

Keranis, E., Makris, D., Rodopoulou, P. et al. (2010). Impact of dietary shift to higher-antioxidant foods in COPD: a randomised trial. *European Respiratory Journal* 36 (4): 774–780.

Lagiou, P., Sandin, S., Lof, M. et al. (2012). Low carbohydrate-high protein diet and incidence of cardiovascular diseases in Swedish women: prospective cohort study. *BMJ* 344 https://doi.org/10.1136/bmj.e4026.

Lee, Y., Berryman, C.E., West, S.G. et al. (2017). Effects of dark chocolate and almonds on cardiovascular risk factors in overweight and obese individuals: a Randomized Controlled-Feeding Trial. *Journal of the American Heart Association* 6 (12): e005162. doi: 10.1161/JAHA.116.005162. PMID: 29187388; PMCID: PMC5778992.

Lianov, L. and Johnson, M. (2010). Physician competencies for prescribing lifestyle medicine. *JAMA.* 304 (2): 202–203.

Lin, J., Hu, F.B., and Curhan, G.C. (2010). Associations of diet with albuminuria and kidney function decline. *Clinical Journal of the American Society of Nephrology* 5 (5): 836–843.

Mayo Clinic (2020). Transfat is double trouble for your heart health. https://www.mayoclinic.org/diseases-conditions/high-blood-cholesterol/in-depth/trans-fat/art-20046114

Mechley, A.R. and Dysinger, W. (2015). Intensive therapeutic lifestyle change programs: a progressive way to successfully manage health care. *American Journal of Lifestyle Medicine.* 9 (5): 354–360. https://doi.org/10.1177/1559827615592344.

Naghshi, S., Sadeghi, O., Willett, W.C., and Esmaillzadeh, A. (2020). Dietary intake of total, animal, and plant proteins and risk of all cause, cardiovascular, and cancer mortality: systematic review and dose-response meta-analysis of prospective cohort studies. *BMJ* 2020: 370: m2412 doi: https://doi.org/10.1136/bmj.m2412.

Narayan, K.M., Boyle, J.P., Thompson, T.J. et al. (2003). Lifetime risk for diabetes mellitus in the United States. *JAMA.* 290 (14): 1884–1890. doi:10.1001/jama.290.14.1884. PMID: 14532317.

National Center for Biotechnology Information (2020a). PubChem Compound Summary for CID 985, Palmitic acid. *PubChem* https://pubchem.ncbi.nlm.nih.gov/compound/Palmitic-acid (accessed 30 December 2020).

National Center for Biotechnology Information (2020b). PubChem Compound Summary for CID 3893, Lauric acid. *PubChem* https://pubchem.ncbi.nlm.nih.gov/compound/Lauric-acid. (accessed 30 December 2020).

Olsen, J.M. and Nesbitt, B.J. (2010). Health coaching to improve healthy lifestyle behaviors: an integrative review. *American Journal of Health Promotion* 25 (1): e1–e12.

Ornish, D., Scherwitz, L.W., Billings, J.H. et al. (1998). Intensive lifestyle changes for reversal of coronary heart disease. *JAMA.* 280 (23): 2001–2007.

Pagona, L., Sven, S., LofMarie et al. (2012). Low carbohydrate-high protein diet and incidence of cardiovascular diseases in Swedish women: prospective cohort study. *BMJ* 344: e4026.

Palmer, S. and Whybrow, A. (2003). Health coaching to facilitate the promotion of healthy behaviour and achievement of health-related goals. *International Journal of Health Promotion and Education* 41 (3): 91–93.

Patel, N., Jayswal, S., and Maitreya, B.B. (2019). Dark chocolate: consumption for human health. *Journal of Pharmacognosy and Phytochemistry* 8 (3): 2887–2890.

Peterson, A.E. and Maryniuk, M.D. (1996). Using a nutrition assessment to determine a nutrition prescription. *The Diabetes Educator* 22 (3): 205-6–209-10.

Pierce, J.P., Stefanick, M.L., Flatt, S.W. et al. (2007). Greater survival after breast cancer in physically active women with high vegetable-fruit intake regardless of obesity. *Journal of Clinical Oncology: Official Journal of the American Society of Clinical Oncology* 25 (17): 2345.

Salt:the facts (2018). https://www.nhs.uk/live-well/eat-well/salt-nutrition/ (accessed 31 December 2020).

Sanchez, A., Mejia, A., Sanchez, J. et al. (2019). Diets with customary levels of fat from plant origin may reverse coronary artery disease. *Medical Hypotheses* 122: 103–105.

Trautwein, E.A. and McKay, S. (2020). the role of specific components of a plant-based diet in management of dyslipidemia and the impact on cardiovascular risk. *Nutrients* 12 (9): 2671.

Tuso, P., Stoll, S.R., and Li, W.W. (2015). A plant-based diet, atherogenesis, and coronary artery disease prevention. *The Permanente Journal* 19 (1): 62.

Uribarri, J., Woodruff, S., Goodman, S. et al. (2010). Advanced glycation end products in foods and a practical guide to their reduction in the diet. *Journal of the American Dietetic Association* 110 (6): 911–16.e12. https://doi.org/10.1016/j.jada.2010.03.018.

Vigneri, R., Sciacca, L., and Vigneri, P. (2020). Rethinking the relationship between insulin and cancer. *Trends in Endocrinology and Metabolism.* 31 (8): 551–560.

Walda, I.C., Tabak, C., Smit, H.A. et al. (2002). Diet and 20-year chronic obstructive pulmonary disease mortality in middle-aged men from three European countries. *European Journal of Clinical Nutrition* 56 (7): 638–643.

Yokoyama, Y., Levin, S.M., and Barnard, N.D. (2017). Association between plant-based diets and plasma lipids: a systematic review and meta-analysis. *Nutrition Reviews* 75 (9): 683–698.

CHAPTER 6

Physical Activity Science and Prescription

Introduction

Physical activity is a cornerstone of lifestyle medicine and lack of it is one of the most important modifiable risk factors for lifestyle-related chronic disease. There is good evidence that supports the efficacy of clinician-initiated physical activity counselling, prescription, and referrals to appropriate allied health and fitness professionals. Consequently, physicians are encouraged to use physical activity vital signs and exercise prescription in their practices. This chapter seeks to not only develop an understanding of different types of exercise (including strengthening, aerobic, and stretching), but also exercise intensity, exercise prescription, activity guidelines and counselling, METs, global activity/inactivity levels and measures/scales of activity. Finally, we explore a limited evidence base comparing the effects of medications and physical activity on health outcomes. These questions test the candidates on the knowledge and application of exercise and lifestyle interventions in the prevention, treatment, and reversal of inactivity on chronic lifestyle-related diseases.

1. Flexibility is best characterized by:
   a. Increased flexibility of most joints through exercise
   b. Excessive range of movement associated with risk of injury
   c. Reduced range of motion
   d. Stretchy skin, scarring and joint dislocation

Lifestyle Medicine: Essential MCQs for Certification in Lifestyle Medicine, First Edition.
Ifeoma Monye, Adaeze Ifezulike, Karen Adamson and Fraser Birrell.
© 2022 John Wiley & Sons Ltd. Published 2022 by John Wiley & Sons Ltd.

2. Which of the following best describes the factors determining flexibility at a joint?
    a. Bone alignment, body mass index, waist-hip ratio
    b. Ligaments, muscle tightness, bone alignment
    c. Ligaments, muscle tightness, tendons
    d. Ligaments, skin thickness, oesophageal dysmotility

3. Which would be the most appropriate advice for a patient starting flexibility training?
    a. Bounce frequently after stretching; warm up before activity
    b. Bounce frequently after stretching; hold the stretch for 20–30 seconds
    c. Do maximal stretches from the outset; hold the stretch for 20–30 seconds
    d. Stretch to the point of feeling a tightness in the muscle; warm up before activity

4. Stretching exercises can be done to maintain:
    a. Cardiovascular fitness, slow fibre contractility
    b. Posture, core stability, adrenaline
    c. Power, stability, rehabilitation
    d. Suppleness, range of motion, endorphin levels

5. Which of the following best describes the effects of warming up prior to physical activity (PA)?
    a. Decrease range of motion at a joint, increase physical work capacity, increase the rate of energy release from the body
    b. Increase range of motion at a joint, decrease physical work capacity, increase the rate of energy release from the body
    c. Increase range of motion at a joint, increase physical work capacity, decrease the rate of energy release from the body
    d. Increase range of motion at a joint, increase physical work capacity, increase the rate of energy release from the body

6. Which of the following statements best describe(s) balance?
    a. Balance uses no vestibular information, just joint position sense and visual feedback to optimize postural stability
    b. Balance uses no vestibular information or joint position sense, only visual feedback to optimize postural stability
    c. Balance uses vestibular information, joint position sense, but not usually visual feedback to optimize postural stability
    d. Balance uses vestibular information, joint position sense, and visual feedback to optimize postural stability

7. Which statement best describes the effect of fall prevention exercise programs on fall-induced injuries in community dwelling older adults (El-Khoury et al. 2013)?

a. Exercise programmes designed to prevent falls in older adults also seem to prevent severe injuries caused by falls, admissions, and fractures

b. Exercise programmes designed to prevent falls in older adults also seem to prevent admissions and fractures, but not severe injuries caused by falls

c. Exercise programmes designed to prevent falls in older adults also seem to prevent severe injuries caused by falls, but not admissions or fractures

d. Exercise programmes designed to prevent falls in older adults also seem to prevent severe injuries caused by falls and admissions, but not fractures

8. Which of the following best describes the characteristics of physically active physicians (those doing regular aerobics and strength training)?

a. Less likely to practise preventative medicine, change patient behaviour, counsel patients on physical activity, and lead to improved quality of care for patients

b. More likely to practice preventative medicine, change patient behaviour, counsel patients on physical activity, and lead to improved quality of care for patients

c. More likely to practice preventative medicine, change patient behaviour, not counsel patients on physical activity, and lead to improved quality of care for patients

d. More likely to practice preventative medicine, change patient behaviour, counsel patients on physical activity, and lead to reduced quality of care for patients

9. Which of the following best describes examples of balance exercises?

a. Backward walking, brisk walking, heel walking

b. Backward walking, brisk walking, sideways walking

c. Backward walking, heel walking, sideways walking

d. Brisk walking, heel walking, sideways walking

10. Which of the following best describes examples of aerobic exercises?

a. Bicycling, static stretching, swimming

b. Bicycling, running, swimming

c. Bicycling, running, static stretching

d. Running, static stretching, swimming

11. Which of the following best describes the effects of strength training?

a. Uses passive extension to induce muscle contraction, stimulates the development of muscle strength, increases the ability of a muscle to resist force

b. Uses resistance to induce muscle contraction, inhibits the development of muscle strength, increases the ability of a muscle to resist force

c. Uses resistance to induce muscle contraction, stimulates the development of muscle strength, increases the ability of a muscle to resist force

d. Uses resistance to induce muscle contraction, stimulates the development of muscle strength, reduces the ability of a muscle to resist force

12. Which of the following best describes the benefits of strength training?

    a. Improves heart muscle functioning, increases fatigue, increases basal metabolic rate, increases muscle mass

    b. Improves heart muscle functioning, reduces fatigue, increases basal metabolic rate, increases muscle mass

    c. Improves heart muscle functioning, reduces fatigue, increases basal metabolic rate, reduces muscle mass

    d. Improves heart muscle functioning, reduces fatigue, reduces basal metabolic rate, increases muscle mass

13. Which of the following best describes the benefits of post-menopausal strength training?

    a. Improving strength, improving quality of life, improving endurance

    b. Improving strength, moderating quality of life, improving endurance

    c. Improving strength, improving quality of life, moderating endurance

    d. Moderating strength, improving quality of life, improving endurance

14. Which of the following forces are most likely to be used in strength training?

    a. Body weight, free weights, aerobic exercise, machines

    b. Body weight, free weights, isometric muscle contraction, machines

    c. Body weight, free weights, muscle contraction during shivering, machines

    d. Body weight, free weights, muscle stretching, machines

15. Which of the following sets of tests are most valid to assess exercise intensity?

    a. Heart rate, Metabolic Equivalent of Task, perceived exertion, oxygen saturation

    b. Heart rate, Metabolic Equivalent of Task, perceived exertion, torque test

    c. Heart rate, Metabolic Equivalent of Task, perceived exertion, six-minute walk test

    d. Heart rate, Metabolic Equivalent of Task, perceived exertion, whisper test

16. Which of these best describes the 'talk test' for assessing exercise intensity?

    a. Level 1 exercise allows comfortable singing; level 2 allows talking but not singing; at level 3, talking is near impossible

    b. Level 1 exercise allows comfortable singing; level 2 allows talking but not singing; at level 3, quiet talking is just possible

    c. Level 1 exercise allows comfortable singing; level 2 allows talking but not singing; at level 3, talking is near impossible

    d. Level 1 exercise allows fast talking; level 2 allows talking but not singing; at level 3, talking is near impossible

17. When considering an exercise prescription, which of the following best describes the acronym FITT-VP?

    a. Form, Intensity, Time, Type, Volume, and Progression

    b. Frequency, Intensity, Timing, Type, Volume, and Progression

    c. Frequency, Intensity, Time, Type, Volume, and Progression

    d. Frequency, Intensity, Time, Type, Volume, and Progressive

18. Which of the following cardiometabolic factors have an important relationship with the Physical Activity Vital Sign (PAVS)?

    a. Overweight, obesity, hypertension, age

    b. Overweight, obesity, hypertension, high-density lipoprotein levels

    c. Overweight, obesity, hypertension, low-density lipoprotein levels

    d. Overweight, obesity, hypertension, HbA1c

19. Which of these are potential barriers to physician's counselling on exercise?

    a. Physician's personal health ability, counselling effectiveness, lack of clarity who should counsel

    b. Physician's personal health ability, doubts on counselling effectiveness, lack of clarity who should counsel

    c. Physician's personal health ability, doubts on counselling effectiveness, clarity who should counsel

    d. Physician's personal health inability, doubts on counselling effectiveness, lack of clarity who should counsel

20. Which of the following best describes the recommended physical activity (PA) guidelines?

    a. 150 minutes a week of resistance training, 150 minutes a week of moderate-intensity PA, 75 minutes a week of vigorous-intensity PA

    b. 150 minutes a week of resistance training, 75 minutes a week of moderate-intensity PA, 75 minutes a week of vigorous-intensity PA

    c. Twice weekly resistance training, 150 minutes a week of moderate-intensity PA, 25 minutes a week of vigorous-intensity PA

    d. Twice weekly resistance training, 150 minutes a week of moderate-intensity PA, 75 minutes a week of vigorous-intensity PA

21. Which of the following is most true of PA?

    a. Health benefits generally correlate negatively with activity, some activity is better than none, twice-weekly resistance training is recommended

b. Health benefits generally correlate positively with activity, some activity is better than none, twice-weekly resistance training is recommended

c. Health benefits generally correlate positively with activity, some activity is no better than none, twice-weekly resistance training is recommended

d. Health benefits generally correlate positively with activity, some activity is better than none, five times-weekly resistance training is recommended

22. Which of the following is considered the most important change in PA?

    a. Meeting a target of 150 minutes moderate-intensity or 75 minutes vigorous activity at the weekend

    b. Meeting a target of 150 minutes of moderate-intensity or 75 minutes vigorous activity spread throughout the week

    c. Doing some regular moderate or vigorous activity, even if less than 150 minutes moderate-intensity and 75 minutes vigorous activity per week

    d. Achieving 300 minutes of moderate-intensity or 150 minutes vigorous activity per week

23. Which option best summarizes children's physical activity recommendations?

    a. $\geq$60 minutes per day moderate physical activity, weight-bearing activity for bone, mainly aerobic activities

    b. $\geq$60 minutes per day moderate physical activity, weight-bearing activity for bone, mainly anaerobic activities

    c. $\geq$60 minutes per day vigorous physical activity, weight-bearing activity for bone, mainly aerobic activities

    d. $\geq$60 minutes per week moderate physical activity, weights in the gym for bone, mainly aerobic activities

24. Which best summarizes resting, and moderate and vigorous Metabolic Equivalents of Task (METs)?

    a. Quiet sitting is 0 MET, light housework is 3–3.5 METs, cycling at 10–12 mph is 6 METs

    b. Quiet sitting is 1 MET, light housework is 6 METs, cycling at 10–12 mph is 6 METs

    c. Quiet sitting is 1 MET, light housework is 3–3.5 METs, cycling at 10–12 mph is 6 METs

    d. Quiet sitting is 1 MET, light housework is 3–3.5 METs, cycling at 10–12 mph is 12 METs

25. Which of the following best describes the features of Physical Fitness?

    a. Skeletal muscle appearance, endurance, reaction time

    b. Skeletal muscle appearance, endurance, strength

    c. Skeletal muscle appearance, reaction time, strength

    d. Skeletal muscle endurance, reaction time, strength

26. Which risk factor combination has a higher attributable fraction of death than low cardiorespiratory fitness, according to Blair's J. Sports Medicine 2009 study?

    a. Smoking, hypertension, and hypercholesterolaemia combined in men

    b. Smoking, hypertension, and hypercholesterolaemia combined in women

    c. Smoking, obesity, and hypercholesterolaemia combined in men

    d. Smoking, obesity, and hypercholesterolaemia combined in women

27. Which of the following is most accurate when considering Metabolic Equivalents of Task (METs)?

    a. Years of life lost are inversely proportional to METs expended and are independent of ethnicity, sex and weight

    b. Years of life lost are inversely proportional to METs expended and are independent of ethnicity and sex

    c. Years of life lost are inversely proportional to METs expended and are independent of ethnicity and weight

    d. Years of life lost are proportional to METs expended and are independent of sex and weight

28. Which of the following risk factor changes are most likely to cause a decline in the hazard ratio for mortality?

    a. Less MET hours expended per week

    b. More MET hours expended per week

    c. With increasing age

    d. With increased weight

29. Which of the following best describes High-Intensity Interval Training (HIIT)?

    a. Can include bouts of 3s 'all-out' cycling effort, may total ~15 minutes of all-out exercise over two weeks, results are comparable to traditional endurance training for 10% of the time spent exercising

    b. Can include bouts of 30s 'all-out' cycling effort, may total ~15 minutes of all-out exercise over two weeks, results are comparable to traditional endurance training for 30% of the time spent exercising

    c. Can include bouts of 30s 'all-out' cycling effort, may total ~15 minutes of all-out exercise over two weeks, results are comparable to traditional endurance training for 50% of the time spent exercising

    d. Can include bouts of 30s 'all-out' cycling effort, may total ~150 minutes of all-out exercise over two weeks, results are comparable to traditional endurance training for 10% of the time spent exercising

30. When considering physical activity (PA), which of the following is most accurate?

    a. Multiple short bouts of PA are better

    b. Single long bouts of PA are better

c. It is not known if PA is associated with better all-cause mortality rates

d. 'Weekend warriors' have poorer health than sedentary people

31. Which is the best summary of the WHO Global Health Observatory data on physical activity?

    a. High-income countries have half the prevalence of insufficient activity, males are more active than females, older people are less active than the young

    b. High-income countries have twice the prevalence of insufficient activity, females are more active than males, older people are less active than the young

    c. High-income countries have twice the prevalence of insufficient activity, males are more active than females, older people are less active than the young

    d. High-income countries have twice the prevalence of insufficient activity, males are more active than females, older people are more active than the young

32. Which of these best summarizes the health benefits of regular PA among young people according to WHO?

    a. Better cardiovascular and metabolic disease risk profile, enhanced bone health, fewer symptoms of anxiety and depression

    b. Better cardiovascular and metabolic disease risk profile, reduced bone health, fewer symptoms of anxiety and depression

    c. Better cardiovascular and metabolic disease risk profile, enhanced bone health, more symptoms of anxiety and depression

    d. Better cardiovascular and metabolic disease risk profile, enhanced bone health, more symptoms of anxiety and depression

33. According to the World Health Organization (WHO), which of these best describes the correct ranking for physical activity in school-age adolescents from the highest activity to the lowest?

    a. Eastern Mediterranean, Africa/Western Pacific, Europe, Americas, South-East Asia

    b. South-East Asia, Americas, Europe, Africa/Western Pacific, Eastern Mediterranean

    c. South-East Asia, Europe, Africa/Western Pacific, Americas, Eastern Mediterranean

    d. South-East Asia, Europe, Africa/Western Pacific, Eastern Mediterranean, Americas

34. According to the World Health Organization (WHO), which of these best describes the correct ranking for physical activity in adults from the highest activity to the lowest?

    a. Americas, Eastern Mediterranean, Europe, Africa, South-East Asia, Western Pacific

    b. South-East Asia, Americas, Europe, Africa/Western Pacific, Eastern Mediterranean

    c. Western Pacific, Africa, Europe, South-East Asia, Americas, Eastern Mediterranean

    d. Western Pacific, Africa, Europe, South-East Asia, Eastern Mediterranean, Americas

35. Which of the following best describes the findings of Van der Ploeg et al. in their study 'Sitting time and all-cause mortality in 222 497 Australian adults' (Van der Ploeg et al. 2012)?

    a. An association between sitting and all-cause mortality consistent across the sexes, age groups, body mass index categories, but not physical activity levels

    b. An association between sitting and all-cause mortality consistent across age groups, body mass index categories, and physical activity levels, but not the sexes

    c. An association between sitting and all-cause mortality consistent across the sexes, body mass index categories, and physical activity levels, but not age groups

    d. An association between sitting and all-cause mortality consistent across the sexes, age groups, body mass index categories, and physical activity levels

36. Which of the following best describes the effect of prolonged sitting?

    a. Decrease insulin sensitivity and high-density lipoproteins, enhanced metabolic function, decrease plasma triglyceride levels

    b. Decrease insulin sensitivity and high-density lipoproteins, enhanced metabolic function, increase plasma triglyceride levels

    c. Decrease insulin sensitivity, high-density lipoproteins and metabolic function, increase plasma triglyceride levels

    d. Increase insulin sensitivity and high-density lipoproteins, enhanced metabolic function, increase plasma triglyceride levels

37. As shown by the 'Sitting time and all-cause mortality in 222 497 Australian adults (Van der Ploeg et al. 2012)', duration of sitting time tended to be greater in which groups?

    a. Higher BMI, highest educational levels, rural residence

    b. Higher BMI, low educational levels, urban residence

    c. Higher BMI, highest educational levels, urban residence

    d. Low BMI, highest educational levels, urban residence

38. Which of these best describes the six minutes' walk test (6 MWT)?

    a. The object is to walk AS FAR AS POSSIBLE in six minutes; normal values vary with age, sex, and country

    b. The object is to walk AS FAR AS POSSIBLE in six minutes; normal values vary with age, sex, but not country

    c. The object is to walk AS FAR AS POSSIBLE in six minutes; normal values vary with country, but not age and sex

    d. The object is to walk AS NEAR AS POSSIBLE in six minutes; normal values vary with age, sex, and country

39. Which of the following best describes the Borg Rating of Perceived Exertion (RPE)?

    a. It measures physical activity intensity level objectively, corresponds directly to heart rate, and is rated from 6 to 20

    b. It measures physical activity intensity level objectively, corresponds indirectly to heart rate, and is rated from 6 to 20

    c. It measures physical activity intensity level subjectively, corresponds directly to heart rate, and is rated from 6 to 20

    d. It measures physical activity intensity level subjectively, corresponds directly to heart rate, and is rated from 0 to 20

40. Which of these best describes the 'talk test'?

    a. It is a complex way to measure relative intensity of physical activity, doing moderate-intensity activity you can talk, but not sing, doing vigorous-intensity activity, you can't say more than a few words without pausing for a breath

    b. It is a simple way to measure relative intensity of physical activity, doing moderate-intensity activity you can sing, but not talk; doing vigorous-intensity activity, you can't say more than a few words without pausing for a breath

    c. It is a simple way to measure relative intensity of physical activity, doing moderate-intensity activity you can talk, but not sing, doing vigorous-intensity activity, you can't sing more than a few words without pausing for a breath

    d. It is a simple way to measure relative intensity of physical activity, doing moderate-intensity activity you can talk, but not sing, doing vigorous-intensity activity, you can't say more than a few words without pausing for a breath

41. Which of the following best describes ways of measuring physical activity intensity?

    a. Talk test, Rating of perceived exertion (Borg Rating), Target Heart Rate

    b. Talk test, Rating of perceived exertion (Borg Rating), Basal Heart Rate

    c. Talk test, Rating of perceived extortion (Borg Rating), Target Heart Rate

    d. Walk test, Rating of perceived exertion (Borg Rating), Target Heart Rate

42. Which of the following best summarizes the important steps for a counsellor to include?

    a. Ask, abridge, advise, agree, and assist

    b. Ask, assess, advise, agree, and assist

    c. Ask, assess, advise, avoid, and assist

    d. Ask, bridge, comment, develop, and exit

43. The Activity Counselling Trial (ACT) involved encouraging 54 clinicians to incorporate three to four minutes of PA advice to the routine visit of their sedentary patients. Which of these best describes the key findings of the study at 24-months?

    a. VO_2 max significantly improved in both assistance and counselling groups for men and women

b. VO$_2$ max significantly improved in both assistance and counselling groups for men but not women

c. VO$_2$ max significantly improved in both assistance and counselling groups for neither men and women

d. VO$_2$ max significantly improved in both assistance and counselling groups for women but not men

44. Which of the following best describes the findings of the Effectiveness of Physical Activity Advice and Prescription by Physicians in Routine Primary Care cluster randomized trial (Grandes et al. 2009)?

a. No significant improvements were seen in physical activity, but significant improvements in METs and population achieving minimal recommendations

b. Significant improvements were seen in physical activity, but not METs or population achieving minimal recommendations

c. Significant improvements were seen in physical activity and METs, but not population achieving minimal recommendations

d. Significant improvements were seen in physical activity, METs, and population achieving minimal recommendations

45. Orrow et al. (2012) undertook a systematic review and meta-analysis of randomized controlled trials reviewing the effectiveness of physical activity promotion based in primary care. Which of the following best describes their findings?

a. Primary care promotion of physical activity to sedentary adults significantly increased physical activity levels at 12 months, number needed to treat was 12, exercise referral was not supported by the limited evidence

b. Primary care promotion of physical activity to sedentary adults significantly increased physical activity levels at 12 months, number needed to treat was 12, exercise referral was supported by the limited evidence

c. Primary care promotion of physical activity to sedentary adults significantly increased physical activity levels at 24 months, number needed to treat was 12, exercise referral was not supported by the limited evidence

d. Primary care promotion of physical activity to sedentary adults significantly increased physical activity levels at 12 months, number needed to treat was 24, exercise referral was not supported by the limited evidence

46. A systematic review by Garrett et al. (2011) looked at the cost-effectiveness of physical activity interventions in primary care and the community. Which of the following best describes their findings?

a. Walking, exercise groups, or brief exercise advice on prescription delivered in person, or by phone or mail, supervised gym-based exercise classes or instructor-led walking programmes appeared equally cost-effective.

b. Walking, exercise groups, or brief exercise advice on prescription delivered in person, or by phone or mail appeared to be less cost-effective than supervised gym-based exercise classes or instructor-led walking programmes.

c. Walking, exercise groups, or brief exercise advice on prescription delivered in person, or by phone but not mail appeared to be more cost-effective than supervised gym-based exercise classes or instructor-led walking programmes.

d. Walking, exercise groups, or brief exercise advice on prescription delivered in person, or by phone or mail appeared to be more cost-effective than supervised gym-based exercise classes or instructor-led walking programmes.

47. Which of these best describe(s) the findings of the Tai Chi and Postural Stability in Patients with Parkinson's Disease Trial (Li et al. 2012)?

a. The Tai Chi group performed consistently better than resistance-training and stretching groups; were better in all secondary outcomes; effects were sustained for three months after the intervention

b. The Tai Chi group performed consistently better than resistance-training and stretching groups; were not better in all secondary outcomes; effects were sustained for three months after the intervention

c. The Tai Chi group performed consistently better than resistance-training and stretching groups; were better in all secondary outcomes; effects were not sustained for three months after the intervention

d. The Tai Chi group performed no better than resistance-training and stretching groups; but were better in all secondary outcomes; effects were sustained for three months after the intervention

48. When counselling for physical activity, which of the following best describes the key points in the assessment process?

a. Frequency, deviation, intensity, and types of behaviours

b. Frequency, duration, integration, and types of behaviours

c. Frequency, duration, intensity, and erratic behaviours

d. Frequency, duration, intensity, and types of behaviours

49. The five stages of physical activity include which of these?

a. Conflict, Planning, Action, Maintenance

b. Contemplation, Permission, Action, Maintenance

c. Contemplation, Planning, Action, Maintenance

d. Contemplation, Planning, Active play, Maintenance

50. When considering interventions to change physical activity self-efficacy and behaviour. Which of the following best describes the most effective techniques?

a. Action planning, reinforcing effort towards behaviour, relapse prevention and setting graded tasks

b. Action planning, reinforcing effort towards behaviour, but not relapse prevention or setting graded tasks

    c. Action planning, but not reinforcing effort towards behaviour, relapse prevention or setting graded tasks

    d. Action planning, provide instruction and reinforcing effort towards behaviour, relapse prevention, but not setting graded tasks

51. Which of the following best describes moderate-intensity exercise?

    a. Carrying moderate loads ($< 20\,$kg), hiking, vacuuming the house

    b. Carrying moderate loads ($< 20\,$kg), hiking, volleyball

    c. Carrying moderate loads ($< 20\,$kg), vacuuming the house, volleyball

    d. Hiking, vacuuming the house, volleyball

52. Which of the following statements about Metabolic Equivalents of Task (METs) is most accurate?

    a. METs are not confounded by obesity, reflect individual basal metabolic rate, one MET is the energy cost of sitting quietly

    b. METs are confounded by obesity, reflect individual basal metabolic rate, one MET is the energy cost of sitting quietly

    c. METs are confounded by obesity, do not reflect individual basal metabolic rate, one MET is the energy cost of sitting quietly

    d. METs are confounded by obesity, reflect individual basal metabolic rate, two METs are the energy cost of sitting quietly

53. According to WHO, which of these best describes vigorous-intensity exercise?

    a. Carrying loads $< 20\,$kg, digging ditches, dancing, running

    b. Carrying loads $< 20\,$kg, digging ditches, fast swimming, running

    c. Carrying loads $> 20\,$kg, digging ditches, dancing, running

    d. Carrying loads $> 20\,$kg, digging ditches, fast swimming, running

54. Moderate-intensity exercise is best described by which of the following?

    a. Active involvement in games and sports with children, 3–6 METs, general building tasks (e.g. roofing), housework, and domestic chores

    b. Active involvement in games and sports with children, > 6 METs, general building tasks (e.g. roofing), walking up a hill

    c. Active involvement in games and sports with children, 3–6 METs, general building tasks (e.g. roofing), walking up a hill

    d. Active involvement in games and sports with children, > 6 METs, general building tasks (e.g. roofing), housework, and domestic chores

55. Charles, a 45-year-old man, has been consistently playing football for the past four months. What best describes the stage of change he is at?

    a. Maintenance stage

    b. Action stage

c. Preparation stage

d. Contemplation stage

56. Ben leads a sedentary life as a Computer Scientist. He has thought about joining his neighbour to cycle as his neighbour seems to enjoy this a lot. He bought a bicycle three months ago which he is yet to use but intends to before the month runs out. What best describes Ben's stage of change?

a. Pre-contemplative stage

b. Contemplative stage

c. Preparation stage

d. Action stage

57. Ann, a 56-year-old obese schoolteacher, recently lost her colleague to a heart attack. She has decided she will get more physically active and shed some weight to avoid having a heart attack like her friend. Two weeks ago, she bought an exercise bike and has been consistently using it most mornings. What best describes her stage of change?

a. Contemplation stage

b. Preparation stage

c. Action stage

d. Maintenance stage

58. When counselling for physical activity, which of the following best describes the stage at which problem solving is addressed?

a. Assess

b. Advice

c. Agree

d. Assist

59. Which of the following best describes the elements that may be included in the 'assist' stage of PA counselling?

a. A written prescription, printed support materials, self-monitoring tools

b. A written prescription, printed support materials, Internet-based counselling

c. A written prescription, self-monitoring tools, Internet-based counselling

d. Printed support materials, self-monitoring tools, Internet-based counselling

60. Which of the following best describes elements of relapse prevention?

a. Behaviour skills to get back on track, planning for potential lapses, increases self-efficacy and physical activity

b. Behaviour skills to get back on track, planning for potential lapses, reduces self-efficacy and physical activity

   c. Identifying unhelpful thought patterns, behaviour skills to get back on track, increases self-efficacy and physical activity

   d. Identifying unhelpful thought patterns, planning for potential lapses, induces self-efficacy and physical activity

61. Which of these best describes the members of a multi-disciplinary team to help provide counselling on PA and assist in promoting behaviour change?

   a. Coach, Dietitian, Exercise Physiologist, Physiotherapist

   b. Coach, Dietitian, Physical Therapists, Physiotherapist

   c. Coach, Dietitian, Physiatrist, Exercise Physiologist

   d. Coach, Exercise Physiologist, Physiatrist, Physiotherapist

62. Which of the following are key facts from the WHO on physical activity?

   a. Insufficient physical activity is a leading risk factor for cardiovascular disease, cancer, and diabetes; and death worldwide, globally, one in four adults is not active enough

   b. Insufficient physical activity is a leading risk factor for cardiovascular disease, cancer, and diabetes; and death worldwide, globally, two in four adults is not active enough

   c. Insufficient physical activity is a leading risk factor for cardiovascular disease, cancer, and diabetes; and death worldwide, globally, two in five adults is not active enough

   d. Insufficient physical activity is a leading risk factor for cardiovascular disease, cancer, and diabetes; and death worldwide, globally, three in five adults is not active enough

63. Which environmental factors linked to urbanization are most likely to discourage people from becoming more active?

   a. Fear of violence and crime in outdoor areas, lack of parks, sports/recreation facilities, urban drift

   b. Fear of violence and crime in outdoor areas, poor air quality/pollution, urban drift

   c. Fear of violence and crime in outdoor areas, lack of parks, sports/recreation facilities, poor air quality/pollution

   d. Lack of parks, sports/recreation facilities, poor air quality/pollution, urban drift

64. Which of the following best describes the recommended weekly physical activity for older adults?

   a. The same as all adults, but those with poor mobility should perform physical activity to enhance balance and prevent falls, one day per week.

   b. The same as all adults, but those with poor mobility should perform physical activity to enhance balance and prevent falls, three or more days per week.

c. The same as all adults, but those with poor mobility should also perform physical activity to enhance balance and prevent falls, five days per week.

d. The same as all adults, but those with poor mobility should also perform physical activity to enhance balance and prevent falls, seven days per week.

65. Which of the following statements is most accurate when describing physical activity in older adults?

a. Screening is crucial before older adults engage in regular physical activity

b. Older adults with exertional chest pain do not need to consult a doctor before starting physical activity

c. Palpitations or dizziness prompted by exercise should be discussed with a physician before engaging in mild activity

d. Joint pain is a contraindication for mild physical activity

66. Victor, a 62-year-old man, had a myocardial infarction six weeks ago and received coronary artery stenting. His latest exercise tolerance testing (ETT) was normal. He has stopped smoking. He is keen to change his sedentary lifestyle and has been taking walks around the neighbourhood. His 23-year-old son is a keen runner and has been asking him to join him. Which of the following is the best next step?

a. Refer him for physiotherapy input to tailor an exercise regime

b. Write to his cardiologist and seek an opinion

c. Advise him to start gradually and then build up to the recommended physical activity level of 150 minutes moderate-intensity exercise per week.

d. Advise against regular exercise until six months post infarct

67. In their 2013 study, comparative effectiveness of exercise and drug interventions on mortality outcomes, Naci and Ioannidis, which of the following best describes their findings for physical activity?

a. Physical activity was better than drugs for coronary heart disease and pre-diabetes; equivalent to drugs for stroke; less effective than drugs for heart failure

b. Physical activity was equivalent to drugs for coronary heart disease and pre-diabetes; better than drugs for stroke; less effective than drugs for heart failure

c. Physical activity was equivalent to drugs for coronary heart disease and pre-diabetes; better than drugs for stroke and heart failure

d. Physical activity was equivalent to drugs for coronary heart disease and pre-diabetes; less effective than drugs for heart failure and stroke

68. Naci and Ioannidis (2013) showed more benefit from medication than physical activity in certain conditions. Which of the following best fits their findings?

a. Stroke

b. Coronary heart disease

   c. Pre-diabetes

   d. Heart failure

69. Which of the following best describes the most important steps in physical activity for older adults?

   a. Eat less and move more

   b. Eat less and sit more

   c. Sit less and eat more

   d. Sit less and move more

70. Which of the following statements is most accurate with regard to weight loss and exercise?

   a. People always need more than the recommended 150 minutes' moderate-intensity physical activity per week to lose weight

   b. People vary in the amount of physical activity they need to achieve and maintain a healthy weight

   c. High levels of physical activity alone are required to lose weight

   d. More than 300 minutes per week of moderate-intensity physical activity are the main strategy to lose more than 5% of their body weight

71. Which of the following statements is/are most accurate?

   a. Muscle quality is more important than muscle mass

   b. Muscle quality is improved by intramuscular fat

   c. Muscle mass is more important than muscle quality

   d. Muscle mass is the same as muscle quality

72. Which of these most accurately describes the recommendations regarding physical activity in pregnancy?

   a. In normal healthy women, the recommendation is at least 75 minutes of moderate-intensity aerobic activity per week

   b. Guidelines generally rule out sports with risks of falls, trauma, or collisions

   c. All pregnant women once confirmed pregnant should avoid PA that involves lying on their back

   d. Scuba diving is usually recommended

73. Melanie, a 34-year primiparous woman with well-controlled type I diabetes, develops persistent bleeding at 28 weeks. What would be the best advice regarding physical activity?

   a. Exercise is absolutely contraindicated

   b. Exercise is relatively contraindicated

   c. Light and moderate exercises are recommended

   d. All exercise is safe

74. Which of these is the most accurate about physical activity and prevention of Ischaemic Heart Disease?

    a. In people who already have IHD, further risk can be decreased up to 90% by being active

    b. Minimum recommendation is 150 mins/week moderate-intensity PA

    c. There is limited evidence that PA limits risk of IHD

    d. 75 minutes per week of low-intensity PA is recommended to avoid straining their hearts

75. Which of the following best describes the finding of Choi et al. in their study 'The effects of physical activity (PA) and PA plus diet interventions on body weight in over-weight or obese women who are pregnant or in postpartum'?

    a. Pregnant women in exercise groups gained 0.91 kg less; postpartum they lost significantly more body weight; supervised PA plus diet intervention most effective

    b. Pregnant women in exercise groups gained 9.1 kg less; postpartum they lost significantly more body weight; supervised PA plus diet intervention most effective

    c. Pregnant women in exercise groups gained 0.91 kg less; postpartum they lost significantly less body weight; supervised PA plus diet intervention most effective

    d. Pregnant women in exercise groups gained 0.91 kg less; postpartum they lost significantly more body weight; supervised PA plus diet interventions least effective

76. Which of the following best describes the recommendations on physical activity for people with diabetes?

    a. 150 minutes per week of vigorous-intensity activity

    b. 150 minutes per week of moderate-intensity activity

    c. 75 minutes per week of low-intensity PA

    d. 75 minutes per week of moderate-intensity activity

77. Which of the following best describes the findings of 'Physical Activity of Moderate Intensity and Risk of Type 2 Diabetes: A Systematic Review (Jeon et al. 2007)'?

    a. Regular moderate physical activity and brisk walking gave 30% risk reduction compared to sedentary or next to no walking, respectively in men and women.

    b. Regular moderate physical activity and brisk walking gave 30% risk reduction compared to sedentary or next to no walking, respectively in men but not women.

    c. Regular moderate physical activity and brisk walking gave 30% risk reduction compared to sedentary or next to no walking, respectively in women but not men.

    d. Regular moderate physical activity but not brisk walking gave 30% risk reduction compared to sedentary or next to no walking, respectively in men and women.

78. The results of Physical Activity of Moderate Intensity and Risk of Type 2 Diabetes: A Systematic Review (Jeon et al. 2007) are best described by which of the following?

a. The summary risk ratio for moderate physical activity versus sedentary in type 1 diabetes was 0.69, BMI-adjusted risk ratio was 0.83

b. The summary risk ratio for moderate physical activity versus sedentary in type 2 diabetes was 0.30, BMI-adjusted risk ratio was 0.83

c. The summary risk ratio for moderate physical activity versus sedentary in type 2 diabetes was 0.69, BMI-adjusted risk ratio was 0.83

d. The summary risk ratio for moderate physical activity versus sedentary in type 2 diabetes was 0.69, BMI-adjusted risk ratio was 0.30

79. Reduction in the incidence of type 2 diabetes with lifestyle intervention or metformin (Knowler et al. 2002) showed what?

a. Lifestyle changes and metformin both equally reduced the incidence of diabetes

b. Metformin reduced the incidence of type 2 diabetes by 58%

c. The lifestyle intervention was more effective than metformin

d. The lifestyle intervention reduced the incidence of type 2 diabetes by 31%

80. Which of these statements best summarizes the number needed to treat (NNT) conclusions of Knowler et al. 2002?

a. NNT is the inverse of the absolute risk reduction: 3 persons for three years with the lifestyle-intervention program, and 6 for metformin.

b. NNT is the inverse of the absolute risk reduction: 7 persons for three years with the lifestyle-intervention program, and 14 for metformin.

c. NNT is the inverse of the relative risk reduction: 3 persons for three years with the lifestyle-intervention program, and 6 for metformin.

d. NNT is the inverse of the relative risk reduction: 7 persons for three years with the lifestyle-intervention program, and 14 for metformin.

81. Which of the following best describes the findings of 'Physical activity advice only or structured exercise training and association with HbA1c levels in type 2 diabetes: a systematic review and meta-analysis' (Umpierre et al. 2011)?

a. Structured exercise training with aerobic exercise, resistance training, but not both combined is associated with HbA1c reduction; physical activity advice combined with dietary advice is associated with lower HbA1c

b. Structured exercise training with aerobic exercise, but not resistance training is associated with HbA1c reduction; physical activity advice combined with dietary advice is associated with lower HbA1c

c. Structured exercise training with aerobic exercise, resistance training, or both combined is associated with HbA1c reduction; physical activity advice on its own is associated with lower HbA1c

d. Structured exercise training with aerobic exercise, resistance training, or both combined is associated with HbA1c reduction; physical activity advice combined with dietary advice is associated with lower HbA1c

82. Concerning physical activity and cancer prevention, which of the following is most accurate?

a. There is a dose-response relationship; colon and breast cancer can be reduced by physical activity; activity recommendations are in line with those for all adults

b. There is a dose-response relationship; colon and breast cancer can be reduced by physical activity; activity recommendations are less than with those for all adults

c. There is a dose-response relationship; pancreatic and brain cancer can be reduced by physical activity; activity recommendations in line with those for all adults

d. There is no dose-response relationship; colon and breast cancer can be reduced by physical activity; activity recommendations are in line with those for all adults

83. Which is most true of the effects of increased physical activity on those who have already had cancer?

a. Increased BMI, improved quality of life, decreased peak power output

b. Increased BMI, improved quality of life, increased peak power output

c. Reduced BMI, improved quality of life, decreased peak power output

d. Reduced BMI, improved quality of life, increased peak power output

84. Which of the following best describes the recommended amount of physical activity for disabled patients?

a. Less than other adults

b. More than other adults

c. None unless with another adult

d. The same as other adults

85. The results of 'Tai Chi and postural stability in patients with Parkinson's disease: (Li et al. 2012)' are best described by which of the following?

a. Tai chi training did not affect balance impairments and lowered the incidence of falls as compared with stretching but not resistance training

b. Tai chi training reduced balance impairments and lowered the incidence of falls as compared with both stretching and resistance training

c. Tai chi training reduced balance impairments and lowered the incidence of falls as compared with stretching but not resistance training

d. Tai chi training reduced balance impairments and lowered the incidence of falls as compared with resistance training but not stretching

86. Which statement best describes the effects of physical activity on people living with HIV?

a. Physical activity improved the hemodynamic, biochemical, but not inflamma-tory and immune profile and this effect was not dependent on the use of statins

b. Physical activity improved the hemodynamic, biochemical, inflammatory, but not immune profile and this effect was not dependent on the use of statins

c. Physical activity improved the hemodynamic, biochemical, inflammatory, and immune profile and this effect was not dependent on the use of statins

d. Physical activity improved the hemodynamic, biochemical, inflammatory, and immune profile and this effect was dependent on the use of statins

87. Which of the following best describes the key findings from the Enabling Self-Management and Coping of Arthritic Knee Pain Through Exercise (ESCAPE) knee pain trial (Hurley et al. 2012)?

a. Exercise and education in groups achieved better physical function but higher drug/healthcare/social care costs than usual care sustained for at least 30 months

b. Exercise and education in groups achieved better physical function and lower drug/healthcare/social care costs than usual care sustained for at least 30 months

c. Exercise and education in groups achieved the same physical function and lower drug/healthcare/social care costs than usual care sustained for at least 30 months

d. Exercise and education in groups achieved better physical function and lower drug/healthcare/social care costs than usual care sustained for only three months

88. The benefits of exercise before and after surgery are best summarized as which of the following?

a. Always improves exercise capacity and quality of life

b. Maintained or improved exercise capacity and quality of life

c. Maintained or improved exercise capacity but the worse quality of life

d. Only maintains exercise capacity and quality of life

89. Which statement best describes the effect seen by the addition of video games to early mobilization improving post-operative rehabilitation after coronary bypass surgery?

a. Mixed effects: reduces length of stay and no effect on heart rate variability

b. Mixed effects: same length of stay but improves heart rate variability

c. No: same length of stay and no effect on heart rate variability

d. Yes: reduces length of stay and improves heart rate variability

90. Which timescale best describes how long changes in exercise have been shown to be maintained?

a. At least five days

b. At least five weeks

    c. At least five months

    d. At least five years

91. The effects of exercise therapy on knee and hip osteoarthritis are best described as:

    a. Reduced pain, improved function, performance, and quality of life

    b. Reduced pain and function, improved performance, and quality of life

    c. Reduced pain, function and performance, and improved quality of life

    d. Reduced pain, function, performance, and quality of life

Answers

1. A Flexibility is a feature which varies between individuals, leading to hypermobility where extreme (Birrell et al. 1994) but stretchy skin, scarring, and joint dislocation suggest Ehlers-Danlos syndrome, a group of inherited connective tissue problems. It refers to the range of movement and is increased by exercise (Kelly and Shull 2019, pp. 187–191).

2. C Ligaments, muscle tightness, and tendons are all variables that play a role in flexibility (often referred to as range of motion within the literature; supported by many publications, e.g. Moromizato et al. 2016). Bone alignment affects static position more than flexibility, whereas tendon structure and function are core (think of triggering in flexor tenosynovitis).

3. D There is wide-ranging evidence for flexibility and the role of dynamic (including bouncing) versus static stretching has been explored, for example, in a recent systematic review (Behm et al. 2016). While there is evidence for dynamic stretching, warming up, and stretching technique, there is no current evidence supporting bouncing after stretching.

4. D There are different ways of expressing aerobic exercise, strengthening exercise, balance, and flexibility. Exercise increases endorphins: high-intensity exercise has a bigger effect on these hormones, but moderate-intensity exercise and even stretching still have important effects, explaining why these have positive effects on mood (Saanijoki et al. 2018).

5. D There is strong evidence that warming up has many positive benefits, including the ones listed (e.g. Fradkin et al. 2010; McCrary et al. 2015; Tips Box 6.1).

TIPS BOX 6.1 | Warming Up

- Warming up beforehand improves performance during exercise: improving 79% of outcomes
- Little or no evidence of harm from warming up (Fradkin et al. 2010)

However, not everyone understands and applies the benefits. In a recent Italian survey (Palermi et al. 2020):

- 7% never warmed up
- 77% didn't check their heart rate
- 39% were inactive

Source: –Fradkin et al. (2010) and Palermi et al. (2020).

6. D   Balance integrates information from all these systems, explaining why dysfunction and consequent risk of falling accompany disturbance of any single one (Kelly and Shull 2019, p. 198). Vestibulo-ocular tasks show some promise in improving discrimination post-concussion, compared to vestibulo-spinal testing alone (Moran and Cochrane 2020).

7. A   This systematic review of fall prevention exercise interventions for older community-dwelling people showed improvement with an exercise programme in all four categories of falls were identified: all injurious falls, falls resulting in medical care, severe injurious falls, and falls resulting in fractures (El-Khoury et al. 2013)

8. B   A large study of 1488 primary care physicians in the largest Israeli (1886 791 patients) health maintenance organization examined eight indicators, finding that for all, patients whose physicians were compliant with the preventive practices were more likely ($p < 0.05$) to also have undergone these preventive measures than patients with noncompliant physicians.

9. C   Brisk walking is aerobic exercise, whereas all the others are balance exercises (Kelly and Shull 2019, p. 188).

10. B   Static stretching is not aerobic exercise, but bicycling, running, and swimming are (Kelly and Shull 2019, pp. 188, 198).

11. C   Strength training uses a high percentage of muscle contraction against resistance to maximally stimulate muscle strength and enhance the ability to resist force (Kelly and Shull 2019, pp. 188, 197). A recent systematic review showed resistance training in overweight or obese adults leads to large-strength gains and moderate improvements in physical function (Orange et al. 2020).

12. B   Strength training improves heart muscle functioning, reduces fatigue, increases basal metabolic rate, increases muscle mass (Kelly and Shull 2019, p. 197). A good-sized ($n = 123$) prospective study of a 16-week resistance training programme has shown while adaptation in maximal strength varied by sex, fatigue resistance is independent of sex (Ribeiro et al. 2014).

13. A   Post-menopausal women have the same target exercise as other segments of the adult population, including strengthening, 150 minutes of aerobic and balance exercise (Mishra et al. 2011). Strengthening exercise improves strength, endurance, and quality of life.

14. B   Regular high-intensity contractions at > 80% of maximal power are most effective at improving strength. Forces of this magnitude could come from any of the sources, but stretching, aerobic exercise, and shivering do not create enough load to do so. Although shivering does increase metabolic rate and leads to some release of irisin (Lee et al. 2014), central muscles only achieve 5–16% of maximal voluntary contraction and peripheral muscles only 1–4% (Bell et al. 1992).

15. C Heart rate, Metabolic Equivalent of Task, and perceived exertion are commonly used measures of exercise intensity. Six-minute walk test objectively measures amount of exercise in a standard time period. Therefore, it measures intensity or rate of exercise too. Oxygen saturation is a poor measure of intensity, being affected more by cardiorespiratory issues. Torque test is a homonym for 'talk test'. The whisper test is for hearing (Kelly and Shull 2019, pp. 202, 203, 217).

16. A The talk test is a valid reliable tool for assessing exercise intensity. Level 1 exercise allows comfortable singing; level 2 allows talking but not singing; at level 3, talking is near impossible. It is a practical tool for exercise prescription (Reed and Pipe 2016).

17. C FITT-VP means Frequency, Intensity, Time, Type, Volume, and Progression. These are the characteristics of a systematic and individualized exercise prescription, which is one component to consider in older adults. Other key considerations include pre-exercise screening, considerations for older adults on one or more medications and common barriers to adopting and maintaining exercise in an older population (Zaleski et al. 2016).

18. A In a large recent study, where 50% reported physical inactivity, 26% underactive, and 24% active; younger individuals reported more physical activity. Lower activity groups were significantly less likely to be overweight, obese, or hypertensive, but there was no association with A1c or LDL levels, which are less sensitive to change (Nelson et al. 2020). Intriguingly, a long-term low-carbohydrate diet delivered in groups for type 2 diabetics showed significant improvements in all of these outcomes (Unwin et al. 2019).

19. B Physician's personal health ability, doubts on counselling effectiveness, lack of clarity who should counsel can all impact effective counselling, whereas effective counselling, clarity who does it, and physician's ability are all positives. Recent study showed 'Exercise is Medicine Canada' workshop training can improve practices irrespective of initial confidence levels (O'Brien et al. 2020).

20. D There are consistent recommendations for at least 150 minutes a week of moderate-intensity or at least 75 minutes a week of vigorous-intensity physical activity. Resistance training guidelines vary, but generally recommend at least 8–12 reps for all major muscle groups at least one to two times per week (Fisher et al. 2011).

21. B Health benefits generally correlate positively with activity, some activity is better than none, twice-weekly resistance training is recommended. This is supported by a large amount of evidence, reviewed recently in a systematic review of systematic reviews (Warburton and Bredin 2017).

22. C The review of the reviews challenges current 'threshold-based messaging', concluding that 'the relationships between physical activity and

---

TIPS BOX 6.2 | Physical Activity Recommendations

Children and youth 5–17 years of age should accumulate:

- Average ≥ 60 minutes per day (up to several hours) at least moderate-intensity physical activity
- Some health benefits achieved through average 30 minutes per day
- More vigorous-intensity activities incorporated or added when possible, including activities that strengthen muscle and bone
- Aerobic activities should make up the majority of the physical activity
- Muscle and bone-strengthening activities incorporated ≥ 3 days per week

(Janssen and Leblanc 2010)

Adults should accumulate:

- ≥ 150 minutes of moderate-intensity aerobic physical activity per week
- ≥ 75 minutes of vigorous-intensity aerobic physical activity throughout the week
- Or an equivalent combination of moderate- and vigorous-intensity activities
- Aerobic activity should be performed in bouts of at least 10 minutes' duration
- For additional health benefits, adults can increase moderate physical activity to 300 minutes/week or 150 minutes' vigorous physical activity or equivalent combination
- Muscle-strengthening activities should be done involving major muscle groups on two or more days a week
- Physical activity is for all

Source: WHO (2020a).

---

health outcomes are generally curvilinear such that marked health benefits are observed with relatively minor volumes of physical activity' (Warburton and Bredin 2017).

23. A Recommendations include ≥ 60 minutes per day moderate physical activity, although a very recent systematic review concluded vigorous activity 'may confer greater benefits' (Janssen and Leblanc 2010). They concluded 'aerobic-based activities had the greatest health benefit, other than for bone health, in which case, high-impact weight-bearing activities were required'.

24. C These are respectively examples of resting, and moderate and vigorous activities: Quiet sitting is 1 MET, light housework is 3–3.5 METs, and cycling at 10–12 mph is 6 METs (Haskell et al. 2007).

25. D Physical fitness components skeletal muscle endurance, reaction time, strength, flexibility and body composition. There is plenty of evidence that physical activity enhances mental health (e.g. Wheatley et al. 2020), whereas preoccupation with appearance is a risk factor.

26. A Although low cardiorespiratory fitness was the biggest single risk factor in this study (attributable risk of 16% men and 18% women), combination of hypertension (14% men and 6% women), smoking (8% men and 9% women) and hypercholesterolaemia (3% men and 1% women) exceeds that risk in men but not women (Blair 2009).

27. D While years of life lost is inversely proportional to MET expended and that relationship is consistent across sex and weight categories, African Americans, for example, are at 60% higher risk (Kokkinos et al. 2011).

28. B Mortality increases (and therefore hazard ratio for mortality declines) with each of these apart from increasing exercise measured in MET hours per week, where it decreases (Haskell et al. 2007).

29. B High-Intensity Interval Training can include bouts of 30s 'all-out' cycling effort, may total ~15 minutes of all-out exercise over two weeks, results are comparable to traditional endurance training for 10% of the time spent exercising (Gibbala et al. 2012).

30. A Improvements in all-cause mortality in a large pooled surveillance study in England and Wales were similar for those undertaking insufficiently active participants doing a mean 60 mins per week in 2 sessions, as weekend warriors doing a mean 304 minutes in 1 session. Benefits were intermediate between sedentary and the regularly active group. So little and often was a better strategy (O'Donovan et al. 2017).

31. C There are clear gradients of physical activity across countries, with richer countries having strikingly higher rates of insufficient physical activity (women in Kuwait 75% versus 61% men; WHO 2020a), with higher levels of inactivity for women and older people (although the guidelines for children recommend more, so the prevalence of inactivity values is higher despite this).

32. A WHO highlights the benefits which include better cardiovascular and metabolic disease risk profile, enhanced bone health, and fewer symptoms of anxiety and depression (WHO 2020b).

33. B The relevant adolescent rates of insufficient activity are: Africa 85%, Americas 81%, South-East Asia 76%, Europe 82%, Eastern Mediterranean 87%, and Western Pacific 86% (WHO 2020a). While these are probably tougher questions than you are likely to see in the exam, knowledge and understanding of these gradients for both children and adults will help answering this type of question.

34. D The relevant adult rates of insufficient activity are: Africa 22%, Americas 39%, East Asia 30%, Europe 29%, Eastern Mediterranean 35%, and Western Pacific 19%. (WHO 2020a.) While these are probably tougher questions than you are likely to see in the exam, knowledge and under-standing of these gradients for both children and adults will help answering this type of question.

35. D The association was consistent for all these factors and also for healthy versus those with comorbidities (Van der Ploeg et al. 2012).

36. B Note all these surrogate factors change in an undesirable direction with prolonged sitting (Van der Ploeg et al. 2012).

37. C This is a more nuanced relationship than most where socioeconomic factors drive lifestyle: high BMI, high education (probably a marker of more sedentary white-collar occupations), and urban residence driving sitting, whereas we might expect high BMI, low education, and little rural/urban effect (Van der Ploeg et al. 2012).

38. A These variables all affect 6 MWT, as demonstrated in a multinational comparison across seven countries (Casanova et al. 2011).

39. C This subjective scale was devised by Gunnar Borg and runs from 6-20, where 6 corresponds to a heart rate of 60. The scale is based on the physical sensations that the subject experiences, including increased heart rate, increased respiration or breathing rate, increased sweating, and muscle fatigue (Williams 2017).

40. D This is a revision question to consolidate learning on key features of the talk test (Reed and Pipe 2016).

41. A Talk test, Rating of perceived exertion (Borg Rating), Target Heart Rate (Reed and Pipe 2016; Williams 2017).

42. B The 5 As of counselling are Ask, Assess, Advise, Agree, and Assist (e.g. Vallis et al. 2013).

43. D This sex difference, where VO_2 max significantly improved in both assistance and counselling groups for women but not men, was quite unexpected. Men have much higher baseline VO_2 max and six-month data showed all intervention groups improved (even the advice group), but this was not sustained despite sustained changes in self-report physical activity, again in all groups over 24 months. The authors specu-lated that men might be more responsive to advice, but it is equally likely VO_2 max was not the best primary outcome measure, whereas objective physical activity measurement was more sensitive to change and is a useful surrogate for the long-term outcomes of interest (Blair et al. 1998; ACT 2001).

44. D Significant improvements were seen in physical activity (18 mins/week), 1.3 METs, population achieving minimal recommenda-tions (3.9%; Gonnzalo Grandes et al. 2009). While small, these have population relevance. Secondary outcomes, including cardiorespira-tory fitness and health-related quality of life, were not changed.

45. A Primary care promotion of physical activity to sedentary adults signif-icantly increases physical activity levels at 12 months, number needed to treat was 12 (95% CI 7–33), exercise referral was not supported by the limited evidence (only three trials and a non-significant effect on physical activity; Orrow et al. 2012).

46. D Walking, exercise groups, or brief exercise advice on prescription delivered in person, or by phone or mail appeared to be more cost-effective than supervised gym-based exercise classes or instructor-led walking programmes. Cost-utility was similar to commonly used drugs, supporting wider use of exercise interventions (Garret et al. 2011).

47. A The Tai Chi group performed consistently better than resistance-training and stretching groups; were better in all secondary outcomes; and effects were sustained for three months after the intervention (Li et al. 2012). The outcomes were as good as could be expected and the impressive sustained effects have also been shown in other conditions.

48. D Frequency, duration, intensity, and types of behaviours are all relevant. Other factors include psychological factors such as attitude and self-efficacy (Ronda et al. 2001).

49. C The five stages are Precontemplation, Contemplation, Planning, Action, and Maintenance (Ronda et al. 2001).

50. B Action planning, providing instruction, reinforcing effort towards behaviour were the most effective for changing physical activity self-efficacy and behaviour, but not relapse prevention or setting graded tasks. Counter-productive techniques should be avoided to maximize behaviour change and self-efficacy (Williams and French 2011).

51. A These are all moderate activities apart from volleyball which is vigorous (WHO 2020b).

52. B METs are confounded by obesity, reflect individual's basal metabolic rate, and one MET is the energy cost of sitting quietly (Kelly and Shull 2019, pp. 199, 203, 217).

53. D Carrying loads > 20 kg, digging ditches, fast swimming, running. Carrying loads < 20 kg and dancing are examples of moderate exercise (WHO 2020b).

54. A Active involvement in games and sports with children, 3–6 METs, general building tasks (e.g. roofing), housework and domestic chores are all moderate exercise, whereas walking up a hill and expending > 6 METs are vigorous exercise (WHO 2020b).

55. A This is the maintenance stage (Ronda et al. 2001).

56. C This is the preparation stage (Ronda et al. 2001).

57. C This is the action stage (Ronda et al. 2001).

58. D Assist: Problem-solving occurs at this stage (Meriwhether et al. 2008). Systematic reviews in this area show high-level evidence can and does inform practice (e.g. VanWormer et al. 2009).

59. A   The 'assist' stage could provide the patient with a written prescription, printed support materials, self-monitoring tools (e.g. pedometer, calendar) or Internet-based resources, but Internet-based counselling would be part of the 'arrange' stage (Meriwhether et al. 2008).

60. B   This is a revision of the learning point in question 50 that attempts to prevent relapse are counter-productive, actually reducing the benefits of the intervention including reduced self-efficacy and physical activity (Williams and French 2011).

61. D   All of these have expertise in physical activity and behaviour change, which are the skills needed here; equally a primary care physician can also adopt this role, but a dietitian is more appropriate where nutritional change is needed.

62. A   While each of these estimates on prevalence is true for a country or region, the most recent age-standardized global estimate is 27.5% (95% CI 25–33%), making A the best answer. Note the trend is for increasing inactivity and the confidence limits go from one in four to one in three. So, either one of those would have been the best answer compared to the alternatives presented (WHO 2020a).

63. C   As stated in the WHO fact sheet (WHO 2018), several environmental factors which are linked to urbanization can discourage people from becoming more active, such as fear of violence and crime in outdoor areas; high-density traffic; low air quality, pollution; and lack of parks, sidewalks and sports/recreation facilities. Urban drift describes the movement of rural populations towards cities with industrialization and doesn't directly affect activity.

64. B   Older adults should do the same as other adults: ≥ 150 minutes of moderate-intensity physical activity or ≥ 75 minutes of vigorous-intensity physical activity throughout the week, or an equivalent combination of moderate- and vigorous-intensity activity. For additional health benefits, they should increase moderate-intensity physical activity to 300 minutes per week or equivalent. Muscle-strengthening activities should be done involving major muscle groups, two or more days a week. Those with poor mobility should perform physical activity to enhance balance and prevent falls, two or more days per week (WHO 2018).

65. C   Most people do not need to consult with anyone before regular exercise, but exertional chest pain and potential arrhythmia are two situations when it is recommended to see your doctor first. Once a diagnosis is made, whether of angina or most arrhythmias, exercise is beneficial. Joint pain is also a positive reason to exercise (Roddy et al. 2005).

66. C   Exercise post-infarct does not need to be delayed. He would usually have been offered a tailored post-infarct programme, but self-efficacy and behaviour change are optimized by action planning and patient choice.

67. B This was a meta-analysis of randomized controlled trials with mortality outcomes comparing the effectiveness of exercise and drug interventions with each other or with control. Despite the cost and potential toxicities from drug therapy, no statistically detectable differences were evident between exercise and drug interventions in the secondary prevention of coronary heart disease and prediabetes (Naci and Ioannidis 2013).

68. D The striking finding from this study was how much better physical activity interventions were than drug treatment among patients with stroke: odds ratios, exercise v anticoagulants 0.09, 95% credible intervals 0.01–0.70 and exercise v antiplatelets 0.10, 0.01–0.62 (Naci and Ioannidis 2013).

Heart failure was the only condition studied which improved more with drugs. And although diuretics were more effective than exercise in heart failure, the confidence limits were wide with only marginal statistical significance despite the odds ratio point estimate of 4.11 (95% CI 1.17–24.7; Naci and Ioannidis 2013).

69. D Given the health benefits from reducing sedentary time and doing any exercise rather than none, this analysis piece based on US National Health and Nutrition Examination Survey (NHANES) accelerometry data focused on two key messages: to sit less and move more (Sparling et al. 2015).

70. B Weight loss is achieved by a balance between diet and physical activity with more emphasis on diet. There are more dietary than physical activity interventions showing sustained weight loss, including at the level of ≥ 5% of body weight. So, an understanding that healthy weight can be achieved and maintained with varying levels of activity individuals is the most accurate answer. In particular, one recent review concluded 'unless the overall volume of aerobic exercise training is very high, clinically significant weight loss is unlikely to occur' (Swift et al. 2014).

71. A This is one situation where quality is more important than quantity. For example, strength declines much more than muscle mass in the Health ABC study in this paper already cited over 2000 times (Goodpaster et al. 2006).

72. B Guidelines generally rule out sports with risks of falls, trauma, or collisions. ≥ 150 minutes' moderate exercise is recommended, consistent with all other adult groups. After 16 weeks, supine exercise should be avoided, but scuba diving is not recommended at all (Evenson et al. 2014).

73. A There are few situations where exercise is absolutely contraindicated, but this includes persistent bleeding in the second and third trimesters of pregnancy (Evenson et al. 2014; see Tips Box 6.3).

74. B Favourable lifestyle can reduce risk by up to 50% and there is a wealth of evidence with the biggest improvements from at least 150 minutes of moderate exercise per week (Winzer et al. 2018).

TIPS BOX 6.3 | Physical Activity Recommendations During Pregnancy

Recommendations are as per adults (Tips Box 6.2) except for additional precautions and medical advice in certain situations:

Absolute contraindications

- Persistent bleeding
- Significant cardiovascular disease
- Cerclage, incompetent cervix
- History of fetal growth restriction
- Restrictive lung disease
- Multiple gestation
- Placenta previa
- Preeclampsia, pregnancy-induced hypertension (although physical activity reduces the risk of developing these)
- Premature contractions or labour
- Premature rupture of membranes

Relative contraindications

- Severe anaemia Hb < 100 g/l
- Unevaluated arrhythmia
- Poorly controlled diabetes, hypertension, or thyroid disease
- Morbid obesity (BMI > 40 kg/m^2)
- Heavy smoker > 20/day

Source: Data from Evenson et al. (2014).

75. **A**   The authors concluded 'PA interventions were effective for OW/OB pregnant as well as postpartum women. On average, pregnant women in the intervention groups gained 0.91 kg less (95% CI: −1.76, −0.06) compared with those in the usual care groups. Postpartum women in the intervention groups significantly lost more body weight (−1.22 kg; 95% CI: −1.89, −0.56) than those in the control groups. In the subgroup analyses by PA intervention types, supervised PA plus diet interventions were the most effective' (Choi et al. 2013).

76. **B**   The recommendations for diabetics are the same as the rest of the adult population, so hopefully easy to remember! (Colberg et al. 2016).

77. A These effects were consistent whatever the type of moderate exercise and sex (Jeon et al. 2007).

78. C This builds on the percentage risk reduction in the previous question to ensure understanding of how these relate to risk ratios. Adjustment very rarely leads to increased magnitude of a relationship (Colberg et al. 2016).

79. C The authors concluded, 'The lifestyle intervention reduced the incidence by 58% (95% confidence interval, 48–66%) and metformin by 31% (95% confidence interval, 17–43%), as compared with placebo; the lifestyle intervention was significantly more effective than metformin' (Knowler et al. 2002).

80. B Number needed to treat (NNT) is the inverse of the absolute risk reduction. 'To prevent one case of diabetes during a period of three years, 6.9 persons would have to participate in the lifestyle-intervention program, and 13.9 persons would have to receive metformin' (Knowler et al. 2002).

81. D 'Structured exercise training that consists of aerobic exercise, resistance training, or both combined is associated with HbA1c reduction in patients with type 2 diabetes. Structured exercise training of more than 150 minutes per week is associated with greater HbA1c declines than that of 150 minutes or less per week. Physical activity advice is associated with lower HbA1c, but only when combined with dietary advice' (Umpierre et al. 2011).

82. A A large review concluded 'The evidence for decreased risk with increased physical activity is classified as convincing for breast and colon cancers, probable for prostate cancer, possible for lung and endometrial cancers, and insufficient for cancers at all other sites' (Friedenrich and Orenstein 2002).

83. D A systematic review of physical activity in cancer survivors concluded 'physical activity was associated with reduced BMI and body weight, increased peak oxygen consumption and peak power output, and improved quality of life' (Fong et al. 2012).

84. D Although disabled adults do less physical activity, the goals are the same, but, of course, actual activities and goals should be personalized. The evidence is strong across multiple outcomes (PHE 2018; see Tips Box 6.4).

85. C 'Tai Chi lowered the incidence of falls as compared with stretching but not as compared with resistance training. . . (reducing) balance impairments in patients' (Li et al. 2012).

86. C Physical activity improved the hemodynamic, biochemical, inflammatory, and immune profile, and this effect was not dependent on the use of statins. Indeed statins had some detrimental effects, including a significant increase in fasting glucose ($p < 0.05$) and creatine kinase ($p < 0.05$; Zanetti et al. 2020).

TIPS BOX 6.4 | Physical Activity Outcomes with Strong Evidence for Physical and Cognitive Impairments

Strong evidence:

- Cardiorespiratory fitness
  - Aerobic capacity
  - Walking speed
- Muscular strength and endurance
- Functional skills
  - Gait pattern
  - Falls prevention
  - Balance
- Disease risk and prevention
  - Daily step count
  - Moderate-vigorous exercise time
  - Body composition
- Psychosocial wellbeing and community
  - Physical wellbeing
  - Pain
  - Social development
  - Quality of life
  - Community engagement

Source: Data from PHE (2018).

---

87. B ESCAPE knee pain showed that group exercise interventions for those with clinical evidence of osteoarthritis can be efficient and have sustained efficacy (Hurley et al. 2012).

88. B There is a wealth of evidence exercise around the time of different surgeries, but most of these do not demonstrate survival benefit. For example, a recent systematic review of exercise pre-/post-lung transplant (Hume et al. 2020).

89. D An RCT in Brazil randomized patients to one of three exercise regimes control group, early mobilization group (EMG), or virtual reality group (VRG, differing from early mobilization only by addition of 2 Nintendo Wii games). VRG had a significantly shorter length of stay and both EMG and VRG maintained better heart rate variability (indicating preserved parasympathetic function; Ribeiro et al. 2021).

90. D Long-term follow-up of subjects completing the Cycling against Hip Pain (CHAIN) programme: a six-week cycling and education treatment pathway for people with hip osteoarthritis. All participants were still engaged in at least one physical activity per week and many reported that they had purchased a bike (29%), joined a gym (30%), or cycled regularly (indoor cycling 25%, outdoor cycling 24%). Eighty participants (96%) reported an increase in knowledge of self-managing their symptoms (Wainwright et al. 2020).

91. A A recent systematic review and meta-analysis with data from 77 RCTs (6472 participants) confirmed statistically significant exercise benefits for pain (effect size 0.56, 95% CI 0.44–0.68), function (0.50, 0.38–0.63), performance (0.46, 0.35–0.57), and quality of life (0.21, 0.11–0.31; Goh et al. 2019).

References

ACT: Writing Group for the Activity Counseling Trial Research Group (2001). Effects of physical activity counseling in primary care: the activity counseling trial: a randomized controlled trial. *JAMA* 286 (6): 677–687. https://doi.org/10.1001/jama.286.6.677. PMID: 11495617.

Behm, D.G., Blazevich, A.J., Kay, A.D., and McHugh, M. (2016). Acute effects of muscle stretching on physical performance, range of motion, and injury incidence in healthy active individuals: a systematic review. *Applied Physiology, Nutrition, and Metabolism* 41: 1–11. https://doi.org/10.1139/apnm-2015-0235.

Bell, D.G., Tikuisis, P., and Jacobs, I. (1992). Relative intensity of muscular contraction during shivering. *Journal of Applied Physiology* 72 (6): 2336–2342.

Birrell, F.N., Adebajo, A.O., Hazleman, B.L., and Silman, A.J. (1994). High prevalence of joint laxity in West Africans. *British Journal of Rheumatology* 33 (1): 56–59. https://doi.org/10.1093/rheumatology/33.1.56. PMID: 8162460.

Blair, S.N. (2009). Physical inactivity: the biggest public health problem of the 21st century. *British Journal of Sports Medicine* 43: 1–2.

Blair, S.N., Applegate, W.B., Dunn, A.L. et al. (1998). Activity Counseling Trial (ACT): rationale, design, and methods. Activity counseling trial research group. *Medicine and Science in Sports and Exercise* 30 (7): 1097–1106. https://doi.org/10.1097/00005768-199807000-00012. PMID: 9662679.

Casanova, C., Celli, B.R., Barria, P. et al. (2011). The 6-min walk distance in healthy subjects: reference standards from seven countries. *The European Respiratory Journal* 37: 150–156. https://doi.org/10.1183/09031936.00194909.

Choi, J., Fukuoka, Y., and Lee, J.H. (2013). The effects of physical activity and physical activity plus diet interventions on body weight in overweight or obese women who are pregnant or in postpartum: a systematic review and meta-analysis of randomized controlled trials. *Preventive Medicine* 56 (6): 351–364. https://doi.org/10.1016/j.ypmed.2013.02.021. Epub 2013 Feb 26. PMID: 23480971; PMCID: PMC3670949.

Colberg, S.R., Sigal, R.J., Yardley, J.E. et al. (2016). Physical activity/exercise and diabetes: a position statement of the American diabetes association. *Diabetes Care* 39 (11): 2065–2079. https://doi.org/10.2337/dc16-1728.

El-Khoury, F., Cassou, B., Charles, M.A., and Dargent-Molina, P. (2013). The effect of fall prevention exercise programmes on fall induced injuries in community dwelling older adults: systematic review and meta-analysis of randomised controlled trials. *BMJ* 347: f6234. https://doi.org/10.1136/bmj.f6234. PMID: 24169944; PMCID: PMC3812467.

Evenson, K.R., Barakat, R., Brown, W.J. et al. (2014). Guidelines for physical activity during pregnancy: comparisons from around the world. *American Journal of Lifestyle Medicine* 8 (2): 102–121. https://doi.org/10.1177/1559827613498204.

Fisher, J., Steele, J., Bruce-Low, S., and Smith, D. (2011). Evidence-based resistance training recommendations. *Medicina Sportiva* 15 (3): 147–162.

Fong, D.Y., Ho, J.W., Hui, B.P. et al. (2012). Physical activity for cancer survivors: meta-analysis of randomised controlled trials. *BMJ* 344: e70. https://doi.org/10.1136/bmj.e70. PMID: 22294757; PMCID: PMC3269661.

Fradkin, A., Zazryn, T., and Smoliga, J. (2010). Effects of warming-up on physical performance: a systematic review with meta-analysis. *Journal of Strength and Conditioning Research/National Strength & Conditioning Association* 24: 140–148. https://doi.org/10.1519/JSC.0b013e3181c643a0.

Friedenreich, C.M. and Orenstein, M.R. (2002). Physical activity and cancer prevention: etiologic evidence and biological mechanisms. *The Journal of Nutrition* 132 (11): 3456S–3464S. https://doi.org/10.1093/jn/132.11.3456S.

Garrett, S., Elley, C.R., Rose, S.B. et al. (2011). Are physical activity interventions in primary care and the community cost-effective? A systematic review of the evidence. *The British Journal of General Practice* 61 (584): e125–e133. https://doi.org/10.3399/bjgp11X561249. PMID: 21375895; PMCID: PMC3047345.

Gibala, M.J., Little, J.P., Macdonald, M.J., and Hawley, J.A. (2012). Physiological adaptations to low-volume, high-intensity interval training in health and disease. *The Journal of Physiology* 590 (5): 1077–1084. https://doi.org/10.1113/jphysiol.2011.224725.

Goh, S.L., Persson, M.S.M., Stocks, J. et al. (2019). Efficacy and potential determinants of exercise therapy in knee and hip osteoarthritis: a systematic review and meta-analysis. *Annals of Physical and Rehabilitation Medicine* 62 (5): 356–365. https://doi.org/10.1016/j.rehab.2019.04.006. Epub 2019 May 21. PMID: 31121333; PMCID: PMC6880792.

Goodpaster, B.H., Park, S.W., Harris, T.B. et al. (2006). The loss of skeletal muscle strength, mass, and quality in older adults: the health, aging and body composition study. *The Journals of Gerontology. Series A, Biological Sciences and Medical Sciences* 61 (10): 1059–1064. https://doi.org/10.1093/gerona/61.10.1059. PMID: 17077199.

Grandes, G., Sanchez, A., Sanchez-Pinilla, R.O. et al. (2009). Effectiveness of physical activity advice and prescription by physicians in routine primary care: a cluster randomized trial. *Archives of Internal Medicine* 169 (7): 694–701. https://doi.org/10.1001/archinternmed.2009.23. PMID: 19364999.

Haskell, W.L., Lee, I.M., Pate, R.R. et al. (2007). Physical activity and public health: updated recommendation for adults from the American College of Sports Medicine and the American Heart Association. *Medical Science of Sports and Exercise* 39 (8): 1423–1434. https://doi.org/10.1249/mss.0b013e3180616b27. PMID: 17762377.

Hume, E., Ward, L., Wilkinson, M. et al. (2020). Exercise training for lung transplant candidates and recipients: a systematic review. *European Respiratory Review* 29 (158): 200053. https://doi.org/10.1183/16000617.0053-2020. PMID: 33115788.

Hurley, M.V., Walsh, N.E., Mitchell, H. et al. (2012). Long-term outcomes and costs of an integrated rehabilitation program for chronic knee pain: a pragmatic, cluster randomized, controlled trial. *Arthritis Care & Research (Hoboken)* 64 (2): 238–247. https://doi.org/10.1002/acr.20642. PMID: 21954131.

Janssen, I. and Leblanc, A. (2010). Systemic review of the health benefits of physical activity and fitness in school-aged children and youth. *International Journal of Behavioral Nutrition and Physical Activity* 7: 40. https://doi.org/10.1186/1479-5868-7-40.

Jeon CY, Lokken RP, Hu FB, van Dam RM. Physical activity of moderate intensity and risk of type 2 diabetes: a systematic review. *Diabetes Care.* 2007;30(3):744–752. doi: https://doi.org/10.2337/dc06-1842. PMID: 17327354.

Kelly, J. and Shull, J. (2019). The Lifestyle Medicine Board Review Manual. Section 6: Physical Activity Science and Prescription, 2ee. American College of Lifestyle Medicine.

Knowler, W.C., Barrett-Connor, E., Fowler, S.E. et al. (2002). Reduction in the incidence of type 2 diabetes with lifestyle intervention or metformin. *The New England Journal of Medicine* 346 (6): 393–403. https://doi.org/10.1056/NEJMoa012512. PMID: 11832527; PMCID: PMC1370926.

Kokkinos, P., Sheriff, H., and Kheirbek, R. (2011). Physical inactivity and mortality risk. *Cardiology Research and Practice*: 1, 924945–10. https://doi.org/10.4061/2011/924945.

Lee, P., Linderman, J.D., Smith, S. et al. (2014). Irisin and FGF21 are cold-induced endocrine activators of brown fat function in humans. *Cell Metabolism* 19: 302–309.

Li, F., Harmer, P., Fitzgerald, K. et al. (2012). Tai chi and postural stability in patients with Parkinson's disease. *The New England Journal of Medicine* 366 (6): 511–519. https://doi.org/10.1056/NEJMoa1107911. PMID: 22316445; PMCID: PMC3285459.

McCrary, J.M., Ackermann, B.J., and Halaki, M. (2015). A systematic review of the effects of upper body warm-up on performance and injury. *British Journal of Sports Medicine* 49: 935–942.

Meriwether, R.A., Lee, J.A., Lafleur, A.S., and Wiseman, P. (2008). Physical activity counseling. *American Family Physician* 77 (8): 1029–1136, 1138.

Mishra, N., Mishra, V.N., and Devanshi (2011). Exercise beyond menopause: dos and don'ts. *Journal of Midlife Health* 2 (2): 51–56. https://doi.org/10.4103/097 6-7800.92524.

Moran, R.N. and Cochrane, G. (2020). Preliminary study on an added vestibular-ocular reflex visual conflict task for postural control. *Journal of Clinical and Translational Research* 5 (4): 155–160. PMID: 33029563; PMCID: PMC7534408.

Moromizato, K., Kimura, R., Fukase, H. et al. (2016). Whole-body patterns of the range of joint motion in young adults: masculine type and feminine type. *Journal of Physiological Anthropology* 35: 23. https://doi.org/10.1186/s40101-016-0112-8.

Naci, H. and Ioannidis, J.P.A. (2013). Comparative effectiveness of exercise and drug interventions on mortality outcomes: metaepidemiological study. *BMJ* 347: f5577.

Nelson, V.R., Masocol, R.V., Ewing, J.A. et al. (2020). Association between a physical activity vital sign and cardiometabolic disease in high-risk patients. *Clinical Journal of Sport Medicine* 30 (4): 348–352. https://doi.org/10.1097/JSM.0000000000000588.

O'Donovan, G., Lee, I., Hamer, M., and Stamatakis, E. (2017). Association of "weekend warrior" and other leisure time physical activity patterns with risks for all-cause, cardiovascular disease, and cancer mortality. *JAMA Internal Medicine* 177 (3): 335–342. https://doi.org/10.1001/jamainternmed.2016.8014.

O'Brien, M.W., Shields, C.A., Solmundson, K., and Fowles, J.R. (2020). Exercise is medicine Canada workshop training improves physical activity practices of physicians across Canada, independent of initial confidence level. *Canadian Medical Education Journal* 11 (5): e5–e15. https://doi.org/10.36834/cmej.68376. PMID: 33062086; PMCID: PMC7522882.

Orange, S.T., Madden, L.A., and Vince, R.V. (2020:S1836-9553(20)30104-1. doi: https://doi.org/10.1016/j.jphys.2020.09.009). Resistance training leads to large improvements in strength and moderate improvements in physical function in adults who are overweight or obese: a systematic review. *Journal of Physiotherapy*. Epub ahead of print. PMID: 33069607.

Orrow, G., Kinmonth, A.-L., Sanderson, S., and Sutton, S. (2012). Effectiveness of physical activity promotion based in primary care: systematic review and meta-analysis of randomised controlled trials. *BMJ* 344: e1389.

Palermi, S., Sacco, A.M., Belviso, I. et al. (2020). Guidelines for physical activity-a cross-sectional study to assess their application in the general population. have we achieved our goal? *International Journal of Environmental Research and Public Health* 17 (11): 3980. https://doi.org/10.3390/ijerph17113980. PMID: 32512767; PMCID: PMC7313455.

van der Ploeg, H.P., Chey, T., Korda, R.J. et al. (2012). Sitting time and all-cause mortality risk in 222 497 Australian adults. *Archives of Internal Medicine* 172 (6): 494–500. https://doi.org/10.1001/archinternmed.2011.2174. PMID: 22450936.

Public Health England (2018). Physical Activity for General Health Benefits in Disabled Adults: Summary of a Rapid Evidence Review for the UK Chief Medical Officers' Update of the Physical Activity Guidelines. HMSO https://assets.publishing.service.gov.uk/government/uploads/system/uploads/attachment_data/file/748126/Physical_activity_for_general_health_benefits_in_disabled_adults.pdf.

Reed, J.L. and Pipe, A.L. (2016). Practical approaches to prescribing physical activity and monitoring exercise intensity. *The Canadian Journal of Cardiology* 32 (4): 514–522. https://doi.org/10.1016/j.cjca.2015.12.024. Epub 2015 Dec 29. PMID: 26897182.

Ribeiro, A.S., Avelar, A., Schoenfeld, B.J. et al. (2014). Effect of 16 weeks of resistance training on fatigue resistance in men and women. *Journal of Human Kinetics* 42 (1): 165–174. https://doi.org/10.2478/hukin-2014-0071.

Ribeiro BC, Poça JJGD, Rocha AMC, Cunha CNSD, Cunha KDC, Falcão LFM, Torres DDC, Rocha LSO, Rocha RSB. (2021) Different physiotherapy protocols after coronary artery bypass graft surgery: A randomized controlled trial. Physiother Res Int. 26(1):e1882. doi: 10.1002/pri.1882. Epub 2020 Oct 25.

Roddy, E., Zhang, W., Doherty, M. et al. (2005). Evidence-based recommendations for the role of exercise in the management of osteoarthritis of the hip or knee--the MOVE consensus. *Rheumatology (Oxford)* 44 (1): 67–73. https://doi.org/10.1093/rheumatology/keh399. Epub 2004 Sep 7. PMID: 15353613.

Ronda, G., Van Assema, P., and Brug, J. (2001). Stages of change, psychological factors and awareness of physical activity levels in the Netherlands. *Health Promotion International* 16 (4): 305–314. https://doi.org/10.1093/heapro/16.4.305.

Saanijoki, T., Tuominen, L., Tuulari, J. et al. (2018). Opioid release after high-intensity interval training in healthy human subjects. *Neuropsychopharmacology* 43: 246–254. https://doi.org/10.1038/npp.2017.148.

Sparling, P.B., Howard, B.J., Dunstan, D.W., and Owen, N. (2015). Recommendations for physical activity in older adults. *BMJ* 350: h100.

Swift, D.L., Johannsen, N.M., Lavie, C.J. et al. (2014). The role of exercise and physical activity in weight loss and maintenance. *Progress in Cardiovascular Diseases* 56 (4): 441–447. https://doi.org/10.1016/j.pcad.2013.09.012.

Umpierre, D., Ribeiro, P.A., Kramer, C.K. et al. (2011). Physical activity advice only or structured exercise training and association with HbA1c levels in type 2 diabetes: a systematic review and meta-analysis. *JAMA* 305 (17): 1790–1799. https://doi.org/10.1001/jama.2011.576. PMID: 21540423.

Unwin, D.J., Tobin, S.D., Murray, S.W. et al. (2019). Substantial and sustained improvements in blood pressure, weight and lipid profiles from a carbohydrate restricted diet: an observational study of insulin resistant patients in primary care. *International Journal of Environmental Research and Public Health* 16 (15): 2680. https://doi.org/10.3390/ijerph16152680. PMID: 31357547; PMCID: PMC6695889.

Vallis, M., Piccinini-Vallis, H., Sharma, A.M., and Freedhoff, Y. (2013). Clinical review: modified 5 As: minimal intervention for obesity counseling in primary care. *Canadian Family Physician* 59 (1): 27–31.

VanWormer, J.J., Pronk, N.P., and Kroeninger, G.J. (2009). Clinical counseling for physical activity: translation of a systematic review into care recommendations. *Diabetes Spectrum* 22 (1): 48–55. https://doi.org/10.2337/diaspect.22.1.48.

Wainwright, T.W., Burgess, L.C., Immins, T., and Middleton, R.G. (2020). Self-management of hip osteoarthritis five years after a cycling and education treatment pathway. *Healthcare (Basel)* 8 (1): 37. https://doi.org/10.3390/healthcare8010037. PMID: 32059546; PMCID: PMC7151257.

Warburton, D. and Bredin, S. (2017). Health benefits of physical activity: a systematic review of current systematic reviews. *Current Opinion in Cardiology* 32 (1) https://doi.org/10.1097/HCO.0000000000000437.

Wheatley, C., Wassenaar, T., Salvan, P. et al. (2020). Associations between fitness, physical activity and mental health in a community sample of young British adolescents: baseline data from the fit to study trial. *BMJ Open Sport & Exercise Medicine* 6 (1): e000819. https://doi.org/10.1136/bmjsem-2020-000819. PMID: 33088584; PMCID: PMC7547542.

WHO (2018). Physical activity fact sheet. https://www.who.int/news-room/fact-sheets/detail/physical-activity (accessed 29 October 2020).

WHO (2020a). Global health observatory. Prevalence of insufficient physical activity among adults. Data by WHO region. https://apps.who.int/gho/data/view.main.2482?lang=en (accessed 29 October 2020).

WHO (2020b). Physical activity. https://www.who.int/dietphysicalactivity/physical_activity_intensity/en/ (accessed 29 October 2020).

Williams, N. (2017). The borg Rating of Perceived Exertion (RPE) scale. *Occupational Medicine* 67 (5): 404–405. https://doi.org/10.1093/occmed/kqx063.

Williams, S.L. and French, D.P. (2011). What are the most effective intervention techniques for changing physical activity self-efficacy and physical activity behaviour—and are they the same? *Health Education Research* 26 (2): 308–322. https://doi.org/10.1093/her/cyr005.

Winzer, E.B., Woitek, F., and Linke, A. (2018). Physical activity in the prevention and treatment of coronary artery disease. *JAHA* 7 (4) https://doi.org/10.1161/JAHA.117.007725.

Zaleski, A.L., Taylor, B.A., Panza, G.A. et al. (2016). Coming of age: considerations in the prescription of exercise for older adults. *Methodist DeBakey Cardiovascular Journal* 12 (2): 98–104. https://doi.org/10.14797/mdcj-12-2-98.

Zanetti, H.R., Mendes, E.L., Gonçalves, A. et al. (2020). Effects of exercise training and statin on hemodynamic, biochemical, inflammatory and immune profile of people living with HIV: a randomized, double-blind, placebo-controlled trial. *The Journal of Sports Medicine and Physical Fitness* 60 (9): 1275–1282. https://doi.org/10.23736/S0022-4707.20.10838-7. PMID: 33124791.

CHAPTER 7

Sleep Health Science and Interventions

Introduction

Healthy sleep is the anchor for a healthy lifestyle. It helps boost mood and IQ, improve memory and concentration, improve productivity, support weight management as well as decrease the risk of lifestyle-related diseases such as obesity, type 2 diabetes, depression, certain cancers, Alzheimer's disease, and heart disease. In recent years, modern lifestyles are often in direct competition with the need for adequate restorative sleep and the consequences that result from the sleep problems have a basis in lifestyle choices such as poor nutrition, inactivity, poor stress management, environmental factors, and much more. Just as these poor lifestyle choices cause problems with sleep, modification of these lifestyle factors and adopting healthy lifestyle changes can often be the solution, bringing about optimal sleep quality and quantity for health, well-being, and improved productivity.

This chapter tests the candidates on the knowledge and application of sleep science and lifestyle interventions in the prevention, treatment, and reversal of chronic lifestyle-related diseases.

1. A 12-year-old boy is brought to you by his mother with complaints of poor performance in academics, increased irritability, and hyperactivity. Lately, he has been observed to be more aggressive towards his younger sister. Parents are in a happy relationship. He eats well and plays active sports in school. He is well liked, has many friends in school, spends a lot of hours playing computer games in his room with them and is usually the last to go to bed, often waking up in a bad mood after four hours of sleep. He is otherwise fit and well. Which of the following is the most likely reason for his symptoms?

Lifestyle Medicine: Essential MCQs for Certification in Lifestyle Medicine, First Edition.
Ifeoma Monye, Adaeze Ifezulike, Karen Adamson and Fraser Birrell.
© 2022 John Wiley & Sons Ltd. Published 2022 by John Wiley & Sons Ltd.

a. He is suffering from substance misuse

b. He is not getting adequate restorative sleep

c. He is being bullied at school

d. He is being unruly

2. Which of the following statements most correctly describes the amount of night-time sleep required by the age group?

a. Infants require 8–10 hours of sleep

b. Newborns require 10–12 hours of sleep

c. Preschool children require seven to eight hours of sleep

d. Toddlers require 11–14 hours of sleep

3. A 45-year-old schoolteacher presents to the outpatient department with complaints of difficulty with sleep initiation. She says that several hours after she has gone to bed, she finds herself still awake, staring at the ceiling of her bedroom. At waking, she feels very tired but must go to work. Her average sleep time is about four to five hours. Which of the following is the most appropriate recommendation to help her sleep better?

a. Do at least 60 minutes of vigorous-intensity physical activity daily

b. Eat a balanced dinner rich in minerals, potassium, and sodium

c. Eat a high-carbohydrate dinner

d. Reduce night-time exposure to blue light

4. A 52-year-old man is seen at the clinic with complaints of early awakening. He can fall asleep within 10 minutes of going to bed but wakes up after three to four hours to pass urine and thereafter he is unable to go back to sleep. His 60-year-old brother was recently diagnosed with cancer. Which of the following is the most appropriate advice for him?

a. Find ways to reduce night-time worrying and ruminating

b. Keep the bedroom lights cool blue to provide a conducive sleeping environment

c. Keep the bedroom temperature warm with the heating on

d. Start taking sleeping pills to see if this helps

5. Which of the following best describes what happens to brain cells during sleep?

a. The brain synapses remain the same

b. The brain synapses double in numbers

c. The brain synapses enlarge in size

d. The brain synapses shrink in size

6. Sleep is important for memory consolidation. Which of the following is the best advice for a 20-year-old student who is struggling to stay asleep and at best gets four to five hours of sleep every night?

   a. Have daytime naps of at least two hours

   b. Have a cup of black tea in the evenings

   c. Have an early morning exercise regimen

   d. Have a prescription for sleeping pills

7. A 75-year-old cohort study on adult development looked at 268 male Harvard students from graduating years 1939–1944 and 456 men from inner city Boston. Which of the following conclusions was reached as the single most important predictor of happiness and longevity?

   a. Having adequate restorative sleep

   b. Having highly nutritious meals

   c. Having social connections

   d. Having an active life

8. Which of the following best represents a consequence of short-term sleep deprivation?

   a. Increased alertness

   b. Reduced levels of stress hormones

   c. Raised blood pressure

   d. Type 1 Diabetes Mellitus

9. A 30-year-old woman has presented with a history of poor sleep, of six months' duration. Which of the following best describes the effects of sleep deprivation in this patient?

   a. Decreased insulin resistance

   b. Decreased gut permeability

   c. Increased levels of Ghrelin

   d. Increased levels of Leptin

10. A 30-year-old woman with a six-month history of poor sleep complains of increased appetite and unwanted weight gain and asks you what may be responsible for the change in her appetite. Which of the following is the most appropriate explanation for her complaints?

   a. Appetite is controlled by self-will; therefore, she should make up her mind to eat less

   b. Ghrelin hormone reduces with sleep deprivation, causing increased appetite

   c. Ghrelin hormone level rises with sleep deprivation, causing increased appetite

   d. Leptin hormone level rises with sleep deprivation, leading to an increase in appetite

A 40-year-old male banker has been struggling with fatigue. He does not have any known health problems but presents with a lack of energy of six months' duration. There is no other complaint. He has tried all sorts of things in the past, including over-the-counter pills as well as prescribed medications with no improvement. He is now very frustrated as he is struggling to keep up with his work and daily chores.

Further history reveals that he winds down every night by checking his text messages and emails, going on his social media on his phone to catch up on happenings of the day and this lasts for about two hours. He eats his dinner which comprises usually of a takeaway at about 9 pm and has needed an additional evening cup of coffee as he finds that this makes him feel less tired. He describes his sleep as fair.

This history is for Question numbers 11–13:

11. Which of the following is the most appropriate recommendation for him?

   a. Avoid using his phone at least an hour to two hours before bedtime

   b. Begin a routine of physical activity just before bedtime

   c. Increase the dose of sleeping pills for two weeks and review

   d. Take a glass of red wine with dinner

12. He returns for follow-up after three weeks, and despite following the advice above, has made little progress. Which of the following is the most appropriate advice?

   a. Increase the tempo of physical activity from moderate to vigorous

   b. Keep the phone by the bedside and use it as an alarm only

   c. Keep the room lighting dim with blue light

   d. Eat dinner at night between 6 and 7 pm

13. His further lifestyle history reveals that he regularly exercises in the gym just before bedtime, takes a glass of wine with his dinner, showers, and goes to bed. What is the most appropriate recommendation at this point?

   a. Avoid red light around bedtime

   b. Increase physical activity to at least 90 minutes daily

   c. Take two glasses of red wine with dinner

   d. Use 2500 K colour warm lights in the bedroom

14. Which of the following best describes good sleep?

   a. Being able to drop off to sleep within 60 minutes of trying

   b. Waking up and wanting to go back to bed

   c. Waking up at the same time every day without an alarm

   d. Waking up after having had so many dreams during the night

15. Which of the following best describes features of the circadian rhythm?

    a. Artificial light source is not relevant to the body's circadian rhythm

    b. External temperature has a negligible effect on circadian rhythm regulation

    c. The hypothalamus is the organ responsible for synchronizing all the body's clocks

    d. The suprachiasmatic nucleus plays a minimal role

16. Which of the following is the most appropriate statement regarding sleep:

    a. Age does not change sleep patterns

    b. Only severe levels of fatigue impair performance

    c. There is a significant effect with driving if the driver is mild-to-moderately sleep-deprived

    d. We are getting about one hour more sleep than we did 60 years ago

17. Which of the following best describes an action in sleep hygiene for sleep improvement?

    a. Decrease bedtime peripheral cutaneous vasodilation by wearing cooling socks

    b. Establish sleep time but wake time can differ depending on your plan for the day

    c. Have power naps of no more than 30 minutes

    d. Use the alarm clock as the room light

18. Which of the following light colours is best associated with better sleep?

    a. Red light

    b. Ultraviolet light

    c. White light

    d. Yellow light

19. Concerning exposure to early morning light, which of the following best explains its relationship with sleep and health?

    a. Exposure to early morning light has an inverse relationship with good-quality night-time sleep

    b. Research has shown that individuals who are exposed to early morning light had lower body mass indices

    c. Receptors in the retinal photoreceptors that exist in the eye are most sensitive when exposed to a short wavelength blue-green light

    d. Receptors in the retinal photoreceptors that exist in the eye are most sensitive when exposed to long wavelength red light

20. Which of the following most appropriately describes the association between the environment and sleep?

a. Outdoor physical activity has been found to be more beneficial than indoor exercise

b. Regular outdoor physical activity is associated with higher levels of serotonin

c. Researchers have not found any superior health benefits with outdoor physical activity when compared to physical activity indoors

d. The indoor gym halogen light has a better effect on quality of sleep when compared to the morning outdoor light

21. A 38-year-old nurse attends your clinic with complaints of urinary frequency, recent weight loss, and fatigue. She is a night-shift worker. Which of the following is the most useful advice at this time?

a. She is not at increased risk of diabetes

b. She should ideally wear sunglasses while at work

c. She may have better sleep if she wears sunglasses on her way home

d. She has a circadian rhythm that is working optimally

22. Which of the following best represents the level of cortisol in the body?

a. Cortisol level is highest about two hours before waking

b. Cortisol has a diurnal pattern

c. Cortisol level is highest at bedtime

d. Cortisol level peaks about three hours after waking

23. A 24-year-old clerk presents at the clinic with a recent onset of poor sleep. He is unable to fall asleep as soon as he goes to bed and finds that he wakes up after five hours and cannot go back to sleep. You decide to advise him on his sleep hygiene. Which of the following best represents a good sleeping routine?

a. A warm bedroom is better than a cool bedroom

b. Doing vigorous physical activity just before bedtime

c. Having a regular sleep time

d. Sleeping in the weekend to catch up on lost sleep during the week

24. Which of the following best represents the consequences of an irregular sleep schedule?

a. Lower daytime leptin

b. Lower daytime ghrelin

c. Lower night-time glucose levels

d. Ten-fold increased risk of diabetes

25. A 49-year-old truck driver attends your clinic complaining of excessive sleepiness and sometimes uncontrollably nodding off while driving. He has tried to increase the amount of coffee he drinks to keep him awake during his journeys, but this has not helped. He wants to know if this is a serious problem. In responding to him, which of the following is the most beneficial recommendation?

    a. He can continue to drive as this will not cause much disruption to alertness

    b. He can be prescribed a stimulant to keep him awake

    c. He is at risk of serious accidents as this can disrupt performance

    d. He can have coffee to keep him alert while driving

26. Which of the following best describes the physiological effects of coffee?

    a. Blocks adenosine receptors

    b. Decreased sleep latency

    c. Reduced sleep time but not sleep efficiency

    d. Reduced wakefulness

27. Concerning REM sleep, which of the following best explains the contrast between adults and children?

    a. Adults older than 50 spend about 50% of their time asleep in REM

    b. Newborns spend about 50% of their sleep time in REM sleep

    c. REM sleep increases with the growth in brain size

    d. There is no change in REM sleep as a child grows into an adult

28. Concerning the activities of the brain during sleep, which of the following best represents the stages of sleep?

    a. Stage 5: REM sleep

    b. Stage 4: Deep sleep with a combination of theta and delta waves

    c. Stage 3: Deepest sleep, theta waves disappear, and there are only delta waves

    d. Stage 2: Light sleep characterized by delta waves only

29. A 49-year-old man attends your clinic for a review of his chronic obstructive pulmonary disease. He has an underlying heart condition. He admits to having long-term sleep difficulties. On further consultation, he says he does not believe in having set times to sleep and wake up and prefers to enjoy a night out with the lads a few times a week, even though this means several late nights. He talks about having anything from three to four hours of sleep during the week and making up for it at the weekend by sleeping in. Which of the following is the most useful advice to give him?

    a. He can pay back the lost sleep hours of the week by sleeping in at the weekend

    b. His sleep debts can cause cognitive dysfunction

    c. His underlying condition is unlikely to be affected by his sleep pattern

    d. He is not in any danger of early death

30. A 58-year-old woman presents with increasing difficulties staying asleep since she went into menopause some five years ago. She has also noticed a steady weight gain and despite all her efforts to lose weight, she is not losing any significant amount of weight. Her BMI is 38 and BP is 158/96. She asks why she is having all these health challenges. Which of the following is the most appropriate explanation for her obesity?

   a. Sleep deprivation causes an increase in leptin, increased appetite, and weight gain

   b. Sleep deprivation is not related to her weight gain

   c. Sleep deprivation causes increase in Ghrelin but a decrease in Leptin, which, in turn, causes obesity

   d. Sleep deprivation causes a rise in Ghrelin, increased appetite, and obesity

31. A 56-year-old patient is on the Alcoholic Anonymous (AA) programme. Which of the following is the most likely withdrawal symptom to expect?

   a. Decreased REM sleep related to withdrawal hallucinations

   b. Increased night-time sleepiness

   c. Reduction in restful sleep

   d. Sleep without interruptions by numerous awakenings

32. A 52-year-old woman comes to your clinic with complaints of poor sleep. She is unable to initiate sleep and when she finally falls asleep, she finds it difficult to maintain sleep. She has no regular exercise routine but eats healthily. Which of the following most suitably describes the association between sleep and physical activity?

   a. Exercise just before sleep will improve sleep quality

   b. Exercise in fit individuals has been found to decrease stage 4 sleep

   c. Insufficient physical activity is associated with two to four times the likelihood of feeling tired

   d. Vigorous-intensity exercise is required to improve sleep

33. A 60-year-old patient who has suffered from Type 2 diabetes for the past 18 years presents with complaints of poor sleep. She can go to bed and wake up after seven to eight hours, but says she feels tired at waking. Her blood glucose has been poorly controlled lately. Her husband says she continually moves her legs while sleeping, disturbing his sleep. She is very worried about her restless sleep and asks for some understanding of what is happening to her. Which of the following is the most accurate interpretation of her condition?

   a. Blood glucose control in diabetes and sleep have no known association

   b. Her poor glucose control is due to poor adherence and not poor sleep

   c. Restless leg syndrome is an uncommon disorder in Diabetes

   d. There is an increased incidence of restless leg syndrome in Diabetes

34. Which of the following blood laboratory tests is most beneficial in the management of restless leg syndrome?

   a. Chloride

   b. Iron

   c. Potassium

   d. Sodium

35. Which of the following conditions is the best example of a lifestyle-related sleep disorder?

   a. Sleepwalking

   b. Sleep talking

   c. Obstructive sleep apnoea

   d. Nightmares

36. Which of the following conditions best represents a sub-category of a Dyssomnia?

   a. Arousal disorders

   b. Restless legs syndrome disorders

   c. Sleepwalking

   d. Seasonal affective disorder

37. Which of the following conditions is the best example of Parasomnia?

   a. Insomnia

   b. Narcolepsy

   c. Sleep terrors

   d. Sleep apnoea

38. A 30-year-old woman presents with tiredness, a reduced appetite for many of her favourite foods, and poor sleep. Which of the following is least likely to be a possible diagnosis?

   a. Fibromyalgia

   b. Inflammatory bowel disease

   c. Irritable bowel syndrome

   d. Pica

39. Which of the following management approaches will be most appropriate for a patient with chronic insomnia related to lifestyle factors?

   a. Power naps are helpful if they are up to, but no more than, 30 minutes

   b. Sleep medication is the preferred first line of treatment

c. The content and timing of dinner have little or no bearing to management

d. Use a bed for sleep, sex, and reading novels only

40. In the management of chronic insomnia, which of the following statements most accurately represents the best approach to lifestyle intervention?

   a. Cognitive behavioural therapy is highly effective

   b. Medications should be used as first-line treatment

   c. Maintaining a sleep diary is useful only for diagnosis

   d. One day food diary is highly predictive

41. Which of the following statements most suitably describes a feature of obstructive sleep apnoea?

   a. Associated with erectile dysfunction

   b. Incidence is decreasing

   c. Not associated with myocardial infarction

   d. Not found among slim people

42. A 39-year-old schoolteacher who is having a recent challenge at her workplace has presented to you. She is now finding that her sleep is disrupted as she finds it difficult to maintain sleep at night. She comes to you for treatment of her sleep disorder. Which of the following is the most suitable recommendation for her?

   a. Increase morning and mid-afternoon sunlight exposure

   b. Increase physical activity from moderate to vigorous

   c. Sleep in a room that has light curtains to let the evening sun through

   d. Use blue-green-toned nightlights if light is necessary

43. Which of the following best describes features of optimal sleep?

   a. Excessive regular daytime sleepiness is associated with weight loss problems

   b. Having the same routine around sleep has no effect on sleep quality

   c. Less than seven hours can be beneficial to health

   d. More than eight-and-a-half hours can be associated with obesity

44. In prescribing supplemental melatonin for jet lag, which of the following is the most appropriate statement?

   a. Supplementation appears to suppress endogenous melatonin

   b. Supplements can be taken with other supplements with Vitamin B6 with no problems

c. Sustained release preparation may cause morning drowsiness

d. Sublingual preparations do not have better bioavailability than oral tablets

45. A 30-year-old male who is a patient with a known psychiatric illness comes to see you complaining of difficulty falling asleep and staying asleep. Which of the following statements best explains melatonin sensitivity in psychiatric disorders?

a. Patients with bipolar disorder show greater sensitivity to melatonin suppression effects of light at night

b. Patients with seasonal affective disorder do not display any difference to sensitivity to melatonin suppression effects at night

c. Susceptibility to melatonin suppression has no correlation with affective disorders

d. Smoking in psychiatric disorder just before bedtime has not been shown to cause or worsen insomnia

46. Sleep-wake cycle is best characterized by:

a. Circadian rhythm that is determined in the cerebellum

b. Circadian rhythm that is determined by the suprachiasmatic nucleus located in the posterior hypothalamus

c. Homeostatic sleep drive occurring over a period of 24 hours

d. Longer wakefulness leading to reduced drive for sleep

47. A 45-year-old woman comes into the clinic complaining of difficulty concentrating at work of recent onset. She has recently separated from her husband of 20 years and has had problems staying asleep at night. At the end of a hectic day at work, she is exhausted and sleeps off easily but cannot stay asleep, waking up after only three to four hours of sleep and unable to return to sleep. She wonders if she can be prescribed some pills to help her sleep longer as she finds herself struggling through the day with sleepiness, poor concentration, and tiredness. Which of these sleep evaluation options is the most appropriate for her on this visit?

a. Bedtime environment

b. Weekly sleep diary

c. Weekday food diary

d. Weekday exercise diary

48. In the management of insomnia, in a 45-year-old woman, who recently separated from her husband, which of the following is the best course of action?

a. Cognitive behavioural therapy for insomnia is the preferred option

b. Getting back together with her husband is the correct recommendation

c. Pharmacological approach will yield better results

d. Talking therapy will not be beneficial at this time

49. Which of the following most correctly describes the sleep states?

    a. In adults aged 70 and above, the amount of slow wave sleep is the same in both men and women

    b. Non-rapid eye movement stage contains slow-wave sleep

    c. Sleep duration and amount of time spent in each sleep stage remain the same throughout lifespan

    d. Slow wave sleep comprises about 60% of sleep in midlife

50. Regarding normal sleep duration, which of the following best describes associations of sleep duration?

    a. Short duration of sleep is associated with lower daytime Ghrelin

    b. Short duration of sleep is associated with Metabolic syndrome

    c. Short duration of sleep is associated with higher daytime Leptin

    d. Short duration of sleep is associated with reduced intake of carbohydrate-dense foods

51. Sleep duration is best characterized by which of the following statements?

    a. Adults spend about half of their lifetime sleeping

    b. Functional performance is best between 5 and 6 hours/night

    c. Optimal sleep is between 9 and 10 hours for an adult

    d. Short sleep is defined as less than 7 hours/night

52. At sleep onset, which of the following best describes the sleep process?

    a. Excitation of activity in the ascending arousal systems

    b. EEG shows occasional slow waves

    c. There is a decrease in blood pressure and sympathetic tone

    d. There is reduced pineal melatonin secretion

53. Which of the following is the most effective way to review sleep habits in a patient suffering from insomnia?

    a. Sleep diary for the night before the presentation

    b. Sleep diary for the month before the presentation

    c. Sleep diary for the fortnight before the presentation

    d. Sleep diary for the week before the presentation

54. A 55-year-old man attends the outpatient clinic with his spouse who complains that he has restless nights and sometimes stops breathing for a brief moment during his sleep, before resumption of breathing. There is no known past medical history of note. His BMI is 25. In administering the STOP Brief Obstructive Sleep Apnoea assessment tool, which of the following best explains the letters in STOP?

    a. S – Sleepiness during the daytime

    b. T – Tired often

    c. O – Odd breathing

    d. P – Pressure: borderline blood pressure

55. In a meta-analysis of short sleep duration and obesity in children and adults (Cappuccio et al. 2008, which of the following best describes their findings?

    a. Short sleepers had a ten-fold increased risk of obesity

    b. Short sleepers had a four-fold increased risk of obesity

    c. Short sleepers had a two-fold increased risk of obesity

    d. Short sleepers had a seven-fold increased risk of obesity

56. A 40-year-old businesswoman attends your clinic. She has a planned business trip from London to Dubai. She is asking for pills and tips to help her overcome jet lag because she has business meetings from the day after she arrives. She usually suffers from jet lag on that route, feeling very tired and sleepy for the first three days after her arrival. Which of the following is the most appropriate recommendation?

    a. Avoid dim light until one hour before the new ideal sleep time

    b. Get exposure to late afternoon and early evening bright light, preferably outdoors

    c. Get exposure to bright light close to the new ideal wake-up time and preferably outdoors

    d. Take 1 mg of melatonin sublingual three hours before new ideal sleep time

57. In the STOP sleep assessment scores, which of the following is the most accurate interpretation of the assessment tool?

    a. High-risk patients do not require sleep studies, unless there are co-morbidities

    b. Less than three positives equal low risk

    c. T in STOP stands for Targeted Sleep Duration

    d. Two or more positives equal high risk

58. A 60-year-old banker presents with signs and symptoms of snoring, breathing cessation during sleep, daytime sleepiness of six months' duration. You perform a polysomnography. Which of the following is the most accurate interpretation of the apnoea-hypopnoea index (AHI) scores?

    a. Mild sleep apnoea equals less than 5

    b. Moderate sleep apnoea equals 5–15

    c. Severe sleep apnoea equals 30 or more

    d. Severe sleep apnoea equals 15–30

59. About sleep and light exposure, which of the following best describes the association between sleep and light exposure?

    a. Bright sunlight at noon has similar LUX value as bright industrial lighting

    b. Household light is slightly lower LUX value when compared to noon time sunlight LUX

c. Low daytime light intensities significantly increase sensitivity to melatonin suppression from light at night

d. The lower the LUX value, the more the suprachiasmatic nucleus is stimulated to suppress melatonin production and maintain alertness

60. A 66-year-old businessman is travelling from Hong Kong to London. He has made this journey in the past and suffered from jet lag. He now presents to you to prescribe pills and advise him on how to reduce or eliminate jet lag. What will be your best advice?

a. Eat a hearty breakfast within 30–45 minutes after the new ideal sleep time

b. Eat protein-rich dinner two to three hours before new ideal sleep time

c. Get only dim light exposure starting one hour before the new ideal wake-up time

d. Take melatonin timed one hour after the new ideal sleep time

61. A 65-year-old man presents with symptoms suggestive of obstructive sleep apnoea (OSA). You perform polysomnography sleep study. Which of the following most appropriately describes what is measured to chart his sleep cycles?

a. Blood melatonin levels

b. Brain waves

c. Heart sounds

d. Smooth muscle activity

62. A 70-year-old man comes to the primary care clinic with a complaint of difficulty initiating sleep. His bedtime is 11 pm daily. He eats well, does not smoke, does not use recreational drugs, and takes alcohol moderately. He walks his dog every morning for about an hour. He gets into bed at about 11 pm but finds that he really cannot get to sleep for a few hours. He is in retirement but is financially stable and in a good relationship. Which of the following is the most helpful advice for him?

a. Avoid carbohydrate-rich dinners

b. Drink carbohydrate-rich, non-alcoholic fluids with dinner

c. Eat a carbohydrate-rich dinner

d. Eat a protein-rich dinner

63. A 68-year-old man presents with complaints of difficulty in staying asleep. He wakes up to pass urine at 3 am most nights and is unable to go back to bed. Which of the following lifestyle adjustments would be the most appropriate recommendations for the management of maintenance insomnia?

a. Eat an earlier dinner, less salt/spice

b. Eat an earlier breakfast, less salt/spice

c. Eat an earlier breakfast, less salt/more spice

d. Eat an earlier dinner, less salt/no spice

64. A 34-year-old businesswoman is travelling east on a long-haul journey and comes to ask for some advice to combat jet lag. Which of the following is the most helpful advice for her?

    a. Eat a good breakfast within two to three hours of the new ideal wake-up time

    b. Eat a good breakfast within 30–45 minutes of the new ideal wake-up time

    c. Eat complex carbohydrate-rich dinner two to three hours before ideal sleep time

    d. Get exposure to outdoor's bright light just before bedtime

65. For jet lag travelling west, which of the following recommendations is the most relevant to combat jet lag?

    a. Eat a good breakfast two to three hours after the new ideal wake-up time

    b. Eat protein-rich breakfast two to three hours before new ideal sleep time

    c. Eat a good breakfast 30–45 minutes after the ideal wake-up time

    d. Take melatonin 1 mg sublingual at ideal sleep time

66. With exposure to blue light at night, which of the following best describes the physiological effect observed?

    a. Decrease in core body temperature

    b. Decrease in sympathetic tone

    c. Increase in sympathetic tone

    d. Increase in heart rate

67. In advising a new patient seen about sleep hygiene, which of the following will you recommend that they best avoid?

    a. Inconsistent sleep-wake pattern

    b. Increase moderate physical activity to about five times a week

    c. Removal of television from the bedroom

    d. Use of meditation every night to aid sleep

68. A 34-year-old nurse, wife, and mother of two young children, presents with a complaint of early wakefulness of six months' duration. She has no underlying medical condition and she is not on any medication. Lately, her marriage has been difficult as her husband recently lost his job. Angela has tried all she knows about sleep hygiene but there is no improvement. What is the most appropriate advice?

    a. Change bedroom curtains to thick ones that keep out light

    b. Keep a one-month sleep diary

    c. Use your phone alarm and set it at the same time every morning

    d. Stay up late to ensure waking time is pushed back

69. James is a 45-year-old City Executive who presents with a four-month history of poor-quality sleep. He can sleep off easily but finds his sleep is not a deep sleep. He wakes up often and finds it difficult to maintain sleep. He has tried using sleeping pills bought over the counter with no improvement. He does not smoke but drinks wine every night just before bed to help him sleep. Which of the following is best avoided?

a. Alcohol within four hours to bedtime

b. Mid-late afternoon sunlight

c. Mid-late afternoon physical activity

d. Increase in late afternoon hydration with water

70. Monica is a 57-year-old menopausal woman with complaints of difficulties getting to sleep. She has observed that this started a year before her menopause but has worsened in menopause. She has no underlying medical condition, and she is not on any medication. Which of the following is the most appropriate advice?

a. Eat a carbohydrate-rich dinner

b. Ensure regular daily physical activity

c. Use blue light at night in the bedroom

d. Start winding down 10 minutes before bed

Answers

1. B   Chronic sleep deprivation is a common cause of poor educational performance among children of school age. A child with chronic sleep disorder may have learning and memory consolidation impairment at school, irritability and mood modulation alterations, difficulty sustaining attention, and behavioural alterations such as aggression, hyperactivity, or impulsivity (Owens 2008; Hale et al. 2011).

2. D   The National Sleep Foundation recommendations (derived by a multidisciplinary panel) are shown in Tips Box 7.1.

3. D   Sleep initiation disorders are characterized by impairment in the ability to initiate sleep. It is a critical aspect of night-time sleep and must be optimal to ensure restorative sleep. This may occur as a primary disorder or in association with a medical condition. The following are recommendations to help initiate sleep: exposure to early morning sunlight, decrease blue light at night, and bedroom TVs are discouraged for this reason.

TIPS BOX 7.1 | Updated National Sleep Foundation Recommendations

- Newborns (0–3 months): Sleep range narrowed to 14–17 hours each day (previously 12–18 hours)
- Infants (4–11 months): Sleep range widened two hours to 12–15 hours (previously 14–15 hours)
- Toddlers (one to two years): Sleep range widened by one hour to 11–14 hours (previously 12–14 hours)
- Pre-schoolers (three to five): Sleep range widened by one hour to 10–13 hours (previously 11–13 hours)
- School-age children (6–13): Sleep range widened by one hour to 9–11 hours (previously 10–11 hours)
- Teenagers (14–17): Sleep range widened by one hour to 8–10 hours (previously it was 8.5–9.5 hours)
- Younger adults (18–25): Sleep range is seven to nine hours (new age category)
- Adults (26–64): Sleep range did not change and remains seven to nine hours
- Older adults (65+): Sleep range is seven to eight hours (new age category)

Source: Based on Hirshkowitz et al. (2015).

Limit the use of phones to about 90 minutes from the desired bedtime. Avoid physical activity near bedtime (Kelly and Shull 2019, p. 273).

4. A   Sleep disruption can affect the quality and quantity of sleep. The following are recommendations for better sleep maintenance: The bedroom should be at a cool temperature of between 15–19 °C. Avoid extreme temperatures. Red-toned light bulbs are better for aiding sleep. Avoid evening beverages such as caffeine, alcohol, or soft drinks. He is anxious about his brother and, in the first instance, his worries should be addressed (Pan et al. 2012; Kelly and Shull 2019, p. 273).

5. D   Researchers have found that sleep provides time when the brain's synapses shrink back by nearly 20% (Cirelli and Tononi 2017).

6. C   Sleep performs a consolidation and homeostasis that promotes optimal knowledge retention as well as optimal waking brain function. The quality of sleep is vital to understanding how memories are encoded, consolidated, and retrieved. Physical activity, especially in the morning sun, is known to improve sleep quality and quantity (Watson and Buzsaki 2015; Genzel 2020).

7. C   Grant et al. (2015) published a study of adult development and reached the conclusion that social connectedness was the single most important predictor of happiness and longevity (Grant et al. 2015).

8. C   Getting enough sleep is especially important for physical and emotional well-being. Sleep deprivation can lead to many health consequences. There is fatigue, difficulty with concentration, alertness and memory, reduced coordination, raised levels of stress hormones, irritability, increased appetite, and mood changes. Long-term sleep deprivation has been linked to obesity, type 2 diabetes, hypertension, heart disease, and certain cancers (Harvard Medical School Special Health Report 2019); Kelly and Shull 2019, p. 271.

9. C   Two hormones that help regulate hunger are leptin and ghrelin. When the body is sleep-deprived, the levels of leptin fall while ghrelin rises (Kelly and Shull 2019, p. 271).

10. C   Ghrelin stimulates appetite, while leptin decreases it. In sleep deprivation, increased Ghrelin levels and decreased Leptin levels lead to an increase in appetite (Taheri et al. 2004).

11. A   Sleep hygiene refers to habits, behaviours, and environmental conditions as well as other sleep-related factors that can be adjusted as a stand-alone treatment or part of multi-pronged approach in the management of insomnia. Although sleep hygiene has not been found to be effective in all cases of insomnia, many of its components are used with a good outcome in some patients. The sleep hygiene recommendations include exercise, stress management, noise, sleep timing, avoidance of caffeine, nicotine, alcohol, and daytime napping. Others include thinking, planning, and worrying in bed, prolonged periods of non-sleep periods in bed, reading, watching TV, using the phone while in bed, and others. Physical activities should not be done just before bedtime as the body core temperature rises after exercise, making falling asleep difficult. Alcohol may cause drowsiness initially, but this is followed by stimulation. Increasing the dose of medications is ill advised when behavioural approach to management has not been fully explored (Irish et al. 2015; Kelly and Shull 2019, p. 273).

12. **D** Late dinner is associated with difficulties falling asleep and may worsen underlying conditions such as gastric oesophageal reflux disease (Kelly and Shull 2019, p. 273).

13. **D** For optimal sleep, turn off or dim unnecessary lights at least one hour before bedtime. Blue lights, compact lights, halogen lights, and back-lit lights are notorious for contributing to poor sleep. Decrease light at night. Red light promotes good sleep. Use 2500 K-colour warm spectrum lights (red lights; Kelly and Shull 2019, p. 273).

14. **C** Waking up at the same time every day without an alarm shows that the body clock may be working well. The circadian rhythm is best regulated with a healthy habit of having the same sleep and waking times (Kelly and Shull 2019, pp. 261–265).

15. **C** Circadian rhythms direct a wide variety of functions from daily fluctuations in wakefulness to body temperature, body metabolism, and the release of hormones, e.g. growth hormone, leptin, and ghrelin. Circadian rhythms synchronize with environmental cues such as light and temperature (NINDS 2017; Kelly and Shull 2019, pp. 261–265).

16. **C** Sleep patterns change with age. Whereas a newborn requires ~14–17 hours of sleep every day, a teenager needs ~8–10 hours. Adults and young adults need seven to nine hours (Egger and West 2011, p. 227).

17. **C** Bedtime peripheral cutaneous vasodilation should be increased. Regular sleep cycles for bedtime and wake time are crucial for optimal sleep. The alarm clock should be kept out of sight (Kelly and Shull 2019, p. 273).

18. **A** Visible spectrum of light ranges from violet light to red light. Warmer colours like red light support melatonin secretion and promote better sleep (Turner and Mainster 2008; Kelly and Shull 2019, p. 267).

19. **B** Recent research has shown that not getting enough sleep makes you more likely to put on weight (Harvard Medical School Special Health Report 2019).

20. **B** Research findings have not categorically found that outdoor physical activity is superior to indoor physical activity. Evidence in literature suggests that compared with exercising indoors, exercising in natural environments was associated with greater feelings of revitalization and

positive engagement, decreases in tension, confusion, anger, and depression, and increased energy. However, the results suggested that feelings of calmness may be decreased following outdoor exercise. Participants reported greater enjoyment and satisfaction with outdoor activity (Coon et al. 2011).

21. **C**   Her symptoms are suggestive of Type 2 Diabetes. Night-shift workers are at increased risk of Diabetes. Wearing sunglasses at work is not ideal. She has significant disruption of her circadian rhythm (Shan et al. 2018).

22. **B**   Cortisol levels are high in the morning as we wake from a prolonged period of sleep, with an increase of up to 50% in the 20–30 minutes after waking. This is known as the 'cortisol-awakening response' (Kelly and Shull 2019, p. 266).

23. **C**   Sleep hygiene constitutes behaviours and environmental adjustments made to optimize sleep quality and quantity. They include adjustments to sleep regularity, keeping the bedroom at a cool temperature of between 15 and 19 °C, avoiding light an hour before bedtime, avoiding noise, having a bath/shower before bedtime, etc. (Egger and West 2011, p. 236; Kelly and Shull 2019, p. 273).

24. **A**   An irregular bedtime schedule can affect sleep quality and quantity, leading to daytime sleepiness, irritability, and fatigue amongst others. Sleep is regulated by two main processes: the sleep homeostatic drive, influenced by periods of sleep and wakefulness, and the circadian system, an intrinsic pacemaker involving a pathway from the suprachiasmatic nucleus to the hypothalamus. The circadian system has complex interactions with daily behaviours, known as entraining factors. It is thought that having a regular bedtime schedule can strengthen the circadian rhythm; and is beneficial for achieving good-quality sleep. With poor sleep, there is lower daytime leptin and higher daytime ghrelin (Kang and Chen 2009).

25. **C**   Maintaining alertness is critical for the safe and successful performance of most human activities. Microsleeps are particularly concerning in occupations in which public safety depends on extended unimpaired performance, such as truck drivers, locomotive drivers, pilots, air traffic controllers, and process control workers. Excessive uncontrolled naps during continuous vasomotor tasks, such as driving, can be profoundly serious, not only disrupting performance but sometimes leading to injury or death due to accidents (Poudel et al. 2012).

26. **A**   Caffeine causes most of its biological effects via antagonizing all types of adenosine receptors (ARs): A1, A2A, A3, and A2B and, as does adenosine, exerts effects on neurones and glial cells of all brain areas. Caffeine, through antagonizing ARs, affects brain functions such as sleep, cognition, and learning (Ribeiro and Sebastiao 2010).

TIPS BOX 7.2 | The Sleep Cycle: Stages of Sleep

Stage 1: Very light sleep characterized by theta brain waves. This stage is associated with hypnagogic hallucinations (fleeting visual images)
Stage 2: Light/transitional sleep characterized by theta waves with K-complex waves and sleep spindles
Stage 3: Deep sleep with a combination of theta and delta waves
Stage 4: Deep sleep, where theta waves disappear and there are only delta waves
Stage 5: REM (dream) sleep

---

27. **B**   REM sleep decreases with the growth in brain size throughout development, the scientists found. While newborns spend about 50% of their sleep time in REM sleep, that falls to about 25% by the age of 10 and continues to decrease with age. Adults older than 50 spend about 15% of their time asleep in REM (Wolpert 2020).

28. **A**   The sleep cycle: stages of sleep (Egger and West 2011, p. 228; see Tips Box 7.2).

29. **B**   Sleep deprivation is a chronic stressor that causes cognitive problems. This can exacerbate pathways that subsequently lead to disease (McEwen 2006; Egger and West 2011, p. 227).

30. **D**   Healthy sleep quality and quantity lead to lower cortisol and glucose levels, greater insulin sensitivity, higher daytime leptin, and reduced food-seeking behaviours. Conversely, poor sleep will cause lower daytime leptin and higher intake of carbohydrate-dense foods amongst others (Kelly and Shull 2019, p. 271).

31. **C**   Patients on Alcoholic Anonymous (AA) programme can display reduction in restful sleep as a withdrawal symptom (Bayard et al. 2004).

32. **C**   Regular physical activity is beneficial for optimal sleep (Kelly and Shull 2019, p. 273).

33. **D**   There is an increased incidence of restless leg syndrome in Diabetes (Egger and West 2011, p. 232).

34. **B**   There is a clear association between low peripheral iron and increased prevalence and the severity of Restless Leg Syndrome. All patients diagnosed with RLS should have a full evaluation for anaemia (Allen et al. 2013).

35. **C**   In sleep apnoea, a person stops breathing for at least 10 seconds and sometimes for a minute or more. The most common type of sleep apnoea, which has a strong lifestyle link, is obstructive sleep apnoea (OSA; Egger and West 2011, pp. 235–236).

36. B Classification of Sleep Disorders (Egger and West 2011, p. 233).

37. C Classification of Sleep Disorders (Egger and West 2011, p. 233).

38. D Apart from Pica, the rest can present with all the listed symptoms.

39. A Power naps are helpful but should be kept at 20–30 minutes only. Bed should be for sleep and sex only (Kelly and Shull 2019, p. 273).

40. A CBT-I (CBT-Insomnia) has a proven record of accomplishment in the management of chronic insomnia (Clarke et al. 2015).

41. A Obstructive sleep apnoea is associated with erectile dysfunction, obesity, hypertension, heart disease, metabolic syndrome, early morning headaches and diabetes (Egger and West 2011, pp. 235–236; Kelly and Shull 2019, p. 270).

42. A Morning sunlight exposure positively affects melatonin function (Kelly and Shull 2019, p. 267).

43. D The World Health Organization recommends seven to eight hours of sleep every night (WHO 2004), but reverse causation means some obese people sleep longer than normal.

44. C Supplementation of sleep with melatonin can be highly beneficial to sleep deprivation in cases of jet lag (Kelly and Shull 2019, pp. 274–275).

45. A Patients with seasonal affective disorder show differences to sensitivities with melatonin-suppression effects at night (Kelly and Shull 2019, p. 272).

46. C The circadian rhythm is a biological process that regulates the body functions in a rhythm over a period of approximately 24 hours (Kelly and Shull 2019, pp. 262–265).

47. B One of the most effective ways of objectively assessing a person's sleep pattern is by writing down a week's sleep pattern. Mental recall alone is notoriously unreliable (Egger and West 2011, p. 235; Kelly and Shull 2019, p. 276).

48. A CBTI-I is effective for management of insomnia (Clarke et al. 2015).

49. B The sleep cycle (Egger and West 2011, p. 228).

50. B Short duration of sleep is associated with metabolic syndrome. Two hormones help regulate hunger. They are both affected by sleep. When the body is sleep-deprived, the level of ghrelin spikes leading to stimulation of appetite, over-consumption of food and weight gain; while the level of leptin falls leading to an increase in hunger (Taheri et al. 2004).

51. D Adults need seven to eight hours of sleep per night for the best health and wellbeing. Less than seven hours of sleep per night are defined as short sleep duration (Hirshkowitz et al. 2015).

52. C Initiation and maintenance of sleep require suppression of activity in the ascending arousal systems. This happens by inhibitory neurons of the ventrolateral pre-optic area staying active throughout sleep (Carley and Farabi 2016).

TIPS BOX 7.3 | Updated National Sleep Foundation Recommendations

---

Snoring?

Do you **Snore Loudly** (loud enough to be heard through closed doors or your bed-partner nudges you for snoring at night)?

Tired?

Do you often feel **Tired, Fatigued, or Sleepy** during the daytime (such as falling asleep during driving or talking to someone)?

Observed?

Has anyone **Observed** you **Stop Breathing** or **Choking/Gasping** during your sleep?

Pressure?

Do you have or are being treated for **High Blood Pressure?**

Body Mass Index more than 35 kg/m²?

Age older than 50?

Neck size large? (> 16 inches/40 cm measured around Adam's apple)

Gender = Male?

For general population:

OSA – Low Risk: Yes to 0–2 questions
OSA – Intermediate Risk: Yes to three to four questions
OSA – High Risk: Yes to five to eight questions
or Yes to two or more of four STOP questions + male gender
or Yes to two or more of four STOP questions + BMI > 35 kg/m²
or Yes to two or more of four STOP questions + neck circumference 16 inches/40 cm

Source: Based on Chung et al. (2016).

---

53. **D** The prior week's sleep diary, which shows the patterns of sleep, is one of the most effective ways of evaluating the sleep habits of a patient (Egger and West 2011, pp. 231, 235).

54. **B** STOP Brief OSA assessment (See Tips Box 7.3; Kelly and Shull 2019, p. 276).

55. **C** Cross sectional studies from around the world show a consistent increased risk of obesity amongst short sleepers in children and adults (Cappuccio et al. 2008).

56. C Tips for jet lag travelling east: get exposure to bright light, preferably outdoors, close to new ideal wake time, get only dim-light exposure starting one hour before new ideal wake-up time (Kelly and Shull 2019, p. 275).

57. D STOP Brief OSA assessment (See Tips Box 7.3; Kelly and Shull 2019, p. 276).

58. C Polysomnography is the simultaneous recording of brain waves and other measures of physiological functioning to assess sleep (Harvard Medical School Special Health Report 2019).

59. C Low daylight decreases daytime activities, alertness, positive affect, core body temperature. It increases melatonin suppression with evening light (Kelly and Shull 2019, pp. 267, 273).

60. A Conquering jet lag difficulties is still a challenge to many, especially business travellers who need to get into meetings as soon as they arrive at their meeting destinations. A good knowledge of light exposure, food types and timing, and the use of melatonin supplementation is vital to management of this problem (Kelly and Shull 2019, p. 275).

61. B Polysomnography, also called sleep study, is a test used to diagnose sleep disorders. It records the following: Brain waves, skeletal muscle activity, blood oxygen levels, heart rate, respiratory rate, eye movement, and leg movement.

62. A Keep core body temperature down by avoiding a carbohydrate-rich dinner close to bedtime. Some studies have shown that this can delay the onset of sleep. This delaying effect is significantly stronger when carbohydrate-rich foods are consumed close to bedtime (Kelly and Shull 2019, p. 268).

63. A In order to improve staying asleep, the following lifestyle adjustments are recommended: low light before bedtime, more morning light, more afternoon light, earlier dinner, smaller dinner, less salt/spice dinner, more daytime water, less night-time water, no evening caffeine, no afternoon caffeine, minimum/no evening alcohol, mid-afternoon exercise, more physical activity, bedtime calming habit, midnight calming habit, wake-up calming habit, cooler bedroom, and cooler bedding (Kelly and Shull 2019, pp. 267–273).

64. B To manage jet lag travelling east, the following lifestyle adjustments related to meal composition and timing are recommended: eat a hearty breakfast within 35–45 minutes of new ideal wake-up time (Kelly and Shull 2019, p. 275).

65. C To manage jet lag travelling west, the following lifestyle adjustments related to light exposure are recommended: late afternoon and early evening bright light, preferably outdoors, avoid dim-light exposure until one hour before new ideal sleep time (Kelly and Shull 2019, p. 275).

66. C Blue night-time effects increase night-time heart rate, blood pressure, and core body temperature, and decrease sleepiness and suppress melatonin. Blue light creates greater melatonin suppression at lower intensities and shorter durations (Kelly and Shull 2019, p. 267).

67. A Maintaining a regular sleep-wake pattern is vital to optimal sleep (Kelly and Shull 2019, pp. 265, 273).

68. A Shutting out early morning light can aid sleep. Assessing sleep habits requires a week's sleep diary. When the body's circadian rhythm, sleep time, and wake times stay regulated at about the same time, sleep is enhanced (Kelly and Shull 2019, p. 273).

69. B With difficulty maintaining sleep, adjustment is required in the environment (e.g. exclude noise), light (e.g. increase morning and mid-afternoon sunlight exposure), diet (e.g. increase late-afternoon hydration), stress (e.g. mitigate night-time worrying; Kelly and Shull 2019, p. 273).

70. B Regular physical activity especially in the morning is vital for optimal sleep (Egger and West 2011, p. 236; Kelly and Shull 2019, p. 273).

References

Allen, R., Auerbach, S., Bahrain, H. et al. (2013). The prevalence and impact of restless leg syndrome on patients with iron deficiency anemia. *American Journal of Hematology* 88 (4): 261–264. https://doi.org/10.1002/ajh.23397.

Bayard, M., Mcintyre, J., Hill, K. et al. (2004). Alcohol withdrawal syndrome. *American Family Physician* 69 (6): 1443–1450.

Carley, D.W., Farabi, S.S. (2016). Physiology of Sleep.

Cappuccio, F., Taggart, F.M., Kandala, N. et al. (2008). Meta-analysis of short sleep duration and obesity in children and adults. *Sleep* 31 (5): 619–662.

Chung, F., Abdullah, H.R., and Liao, P. (2016). STOP-bang questionnaire: a practical approach to screen for obstructive sleep apnea. *Chest* 149 (3): 631–638.

Cirelli, C. and Tononi, G. (2017). The sleeping brain. In: Cerebrum: The Dana Forum on Brain Science, 07–17. Dana Foundation.

Clarke, G., EL, M.G., Hein, K. et al. (2015). Cognitive -behavioural treatment of insomnia and depression in adolescents: a pilot randomised trial. *Behaviour Research and Therapy* 69: 111–118.

Coon, J.T., Boddy, K., Stein, K. et al. (2011). Does participating in physical activity in outdoor natural environments have a greater effect on physical and mental wellbeing than physical activity indoors? A systematic review. *Environmental Science and Technology* 45 (5): 1761–1772. https://doi.org/10.1021/es102947t.

Egger, G. and West, C. (2011). To sleep, perchance. . . to get everything else right. In: Lifestyle Medicine Managing diseases of Lifestyle Medicine in the 21st Century, 2e (ed. F. Richardson), 226–241. Elizabeth Walton.

Genzel, L. (2020). Memory and sleep: brain networks, cell dynamics and global states. *Current Opinion in Behavioral Sciences* 32: 72–79. https://doi.org/10.1016/j.cobeha.2020.02.003.

Grant, W.T.G. et al. (2015). Study of adult development. http://www.adultdevelopment study.org/grantandglueckstudy (accessed 2 October 2020).

Hale, L., Berger, L.M., LeBourgeois, M.K., Brooks-Gunn, J. (2011). A longitudinal study of pre-schoolers' language-based bedtime routines, sleep duration, and well-being.

Harvard Medical School Special Health Report (2019). Dangers of Sleep Deprivation. Improving Sleep, 1e. Boston, MA: Published by Harvard Medical School. Harvard Health Publishing.

Hirshkowitz, M., Whiton, K., Albert, S.M. et al. (2015). National Sleep Foundation's updated sleep duration recommendations: final report. *Sleep Health* 1 (4): 233–243. https://doi.org/10.1016/j.sleh.2015.10.004. Epub 2015 Oct 31. PMID: 29073398.

Irish, L., Kline, C.E., Gunn, H.E. et al. (2015). The role of sleep hygiene in promoting public health: a review of empirical evidence. *Sleep Medicine Reviews* 2: 23–36. https://doi.org/10.1016/j.smrv.2014.10.001.

Kang, J. and Chen, S. (2009). Effects of an irregular bedtime schedule on sleep quality, daytime sleepiness, and fatigue among university students in Taiwan. *BMC Public Health* 9: 248. https://doi.org/10.1186/1471-2458-9-248.

Kelly, J. and Shull, J. (2019). Sleep science and interventions. In: The Lifestyle Medicine Board Review Manual, 2e, 259–286. American College of Lifestyle Medicine.

National Institute of Neurological Disorders and Stroke (NINDS) (2017). Understanding sleep. https://www.education.ninds.nih.gov/brochures/17-NS-3440-C_508C.pdf (accessed 1 October 2020).

Owens, J. (2008). Classification and epidemiology of childhood sleep disorders.

Pan, L. Lian Z, Lan L et al. (2012). What is the best temperature for sleep?. https://www.healthline.com/health/sleep/best-temperature-to-sleep (accessed 1 October 2020).

Poudel, G., CRH, I., Bones, P.J. et al. (2012). Losing the struggle to stay awake: divergent thalamic and cortical activity during microsleeps. *Human Brain Mapping* 35 (1): 257–269. https://doi.org/10.1002/hbm.22178.

Ribeiro, J. and Sebastiao, A. (2010). Caffeine and adenosine. *Journal of Alzheimer's Disease* 20 (S1): S3–S15. https://doi.org/10.3233/JAD-2010-1379.

Rippe, J.M. (2019). Sleep as medicine and lifestyle medicine for optimal sleep. In: Lifestyle Medicine, 3e. 'Dietary Habits for Sleep Enhancement', 995–1002.

Scully, C.G., Karaboué, A., Liu, W. et al. (2011). Skin surface temperature rhythms as potential circadian biomarkers for personalized chronotherapeutics in cancer patients. *Interface Focus* 1: 48–60. http://doi.org/10.1098/rsfs.2010.0012.

Shan, Z., Li, Y., Zong, G. et al. (2018). Rotating night shift work and adherence to unhealthy lifestyle in predicting risk of type 2 diabetes: results from two large US cohorts of female nurses. *BMJ* 363: k4641.

Taheri, S., Lin, L., Austin, D. et al. (2004). Short sleep duration is associated with reduced leptin, elevated ghrelin, and increased body mass index. *PLoS Medicine* 1 (3): e62. https://doi.org/10.1371/journal.pmed.0010062.

Turner, P.L. and Mainster, M.A. (2008). Circadian photoreception: ageing and the eye's important role in systemic health. *British Journal of Ophthalmology* 92 (11): 1439–1444.

Watson, B.O. and Buzsaki, G. (2015). Sleep, memory & brain rhythms. *Daedalus* 144 (1): 67–82.

WHO (2004) WHO technical meeting on sleep and health. https://www.euro.who. int/__data/assets/pdf_file/0008/114101/E84683.pdf (accessed 30 December 2020).

Wolpert, S. (2020). UCLA-led team of scientists discover why we need to sleep. Health and Behaviour. https://newsroom.ucla.edu/releases/ucla-scientists-discover-why-we-need-sleep.

CHAPTER 8

Emotional and Mental Wellbeing

Introduction

A proper understanding of the relationship between emotional distress and poor health and the role of the health care provider in facilitating patients' emotional wellness is the thrust of this chapter. The presence of co-morbidities will often cause anxiety or depression. Therefore, clinicians should understand the management of anxiety and depression with co-morbidities. Health care providers should be conversant with screening tools for depression and anxiety and be familiar with indications for referral to mental health departments.

This chapter tests the candidates' understanding of the link between emotional distress and health. Key concepts of mindfulness-based stress reduction (MBSR), physician's empathy, and emotional self-management are also tested.

1. Which of these statements best illustrates the relationship between stress and the drive to eat?
    a. Stress has no impact on eating habits or choice of food at all
    b. Stress enhances healthy meal choices due to release of adrenaline
    c. Stressed people more frequently eat nutritious food such as fruits and vegetables
    d. Stressed people more frequently eat palatable non-nutritious food such as fried chips and soda

2. Which of these statements best describes the relationship between stress and health?
    a. A minority of visits to primary care are related to stress and lifestyle
    b. Highly palatable, low-nutrient-dense foods like crisps offer long-term satiety

Lifestyle Medicine: Essential MCQs for Certification in Lifestyle Medicine, First Edition.
Ifeoma Monye, Adaeze Ifezulike, Karen Adamson and Fraser Birrell.

    c. People reporting greater stress most often report greater drive to eat

    d. Stress and weight gain have a consistently negative relationship

3. Which of these options best characterizes symptoms of generalized anxiety disorder?

    a. Decrease or increase in appetite and sleep disturbance

    b. Insomnia, hypersomnia, and irritability

    c. Muscle tension, sleep disturbance, and irritability

    d. Recurrent thoughts of death and eudaimonia

4. Which of these options most appropriately represents diagnostic criteria for depression?

    a. Decrease or increase in appetite and sleep disturbance

    b. Loss of interest in activities that are difficult to do

    c. Recurrent thoughts of death and eudaimonia

    d. Sleep disturbance and irritability

5. The PHQ-4 is an evidence-based ultra-brief screen for Depression and Anxiety. Which of these are features of the PHQ-4?

    a. Feeling courageous or manic

    b. Feeling nervous, anxious, or on edge

    c. Little interest or pleasure in eating

    d. Not being able to stop or control working hard

6. Which of these is true of the PHQ-4?

    a. PHQ-4 does not correlate well with age, employment status, and education level

    b. PHQ-4 has four items screening for depression and eating disorders

    c. PHQ-4 score greater than 2 is a red flag

    d. People with high PHQ-4 should be assessed for suicidal ideation

7. Which of these options best describes non-pharmacological stress management strategies?

    a. Sertraline and mysticism

    b. Tai Chi and SSRI

    c. Tricyclic antidepressants and cycling

    d. Volunteering for meaningful causes

8. Susan, a 44-year-old mother of three children aged between 6, 8, and 10 years, feels constantly overwhelmed. She comes to you tearful and you diagnose mild depression. Which of these would be the most useful lifestyle skill for her to develop?

    a. Avoiding dependence by refusing help from her family and other support network

    b. Isolating herself from mum and children groups as she feels self-conscious

    c. Learning time management skills and relaxation therapy

    d. Making sure she avoids sleeping so she can hear when her children need her help

9. Which of these options is/are key coping skills for the management of stress?

    a. Assertiveness and problem-solving skills

    b. Developing a bitter and sarcastic outlook on life

    c. Learning how to criticize others

    d. Time-wasting skills to delay facing problems

10. Which of these statements best describes relationship between mental health and lifestyle?

    a. Lifestyle medicine tackles the modifiable factors in mental health

    b. Mental illness is usually genetic

    c. Modifiable factors in mental health are lacking

    d. The aetiology of mental illness is straightforward

11. Which of these statements best characterizes the relationship between stress, depression, allostatic load, and diabetes?

    a. Depression is associated with a flatter or blunted diurnal cortisol curve which predicts incident diabetes

    b. Diabetes may predict future depression, but depression cannot predict future diabetes

    c. Studies confirm a unidirectional association only between depression and type 2 diabetes

    d. There is no evidence supporting hypothalamic–pituitary–adrenal axis dysregulation as an important biological link between depression, and type 2 diabetes mellitus

12. Which of these statements best outlines the relationship between coronary artery disease (CAD) and depression?

    a. Modifiable risk factors for CAD include depression, diabetes, and lack of exercise

    b. Persistent generalized anxiety disorder (GAD) but not major depressive disorder significantly increases the risk of incident CAD

    c. Persistent major depressive disorder (MDD) but not generalized anxiety disorder significantly increases the risk of incident CAD

    d. Studies do not support an etiologic and a prognostic role for depression nor anxiety in CAD

13. Joe, a 52-year-old self-employed electrician, is being investigated for angina. He is also moderately depressed with a PHQ-9 of 14 as his business has not been doing too well and his wife has left him. You are considering starting him on antidepressants. Which of these statements is the best clinical course to manage his depression?

    a. An SSRI antidepressant is useful for treating depression in CAD

    b. An SSRI is contraindicated in CAD due to its adverse cardiac effect

    c. An SSRI is safe as it has no effect on the QT interval

    d. Treatment for depression should be delayed until his cardiology appointment in six weeks' time

14. Which of these statements best characterizes the use of tricyclic antidepressants (TCAs) in coronary artery disease (CAD)?

    a. Orthostatic hypotension can be a problem when using TCA

    b. SSRIs prolong QT interval and thus should be avoided

    c. TCAs are generally safer than SSRIs in CAD

    d. TCAs have no impact on the QT interval

15. Which of these statements best summarizes the impact of 'Fast food' and other foods on depression?

    a. During pregnancy, positive correlations are found between fish intake and depressive symptoms

    b. In women, high fish and fresh fruit consumption could increase the risk of depression

    c. Patients with depression who are not suitable for drug therapy or psychotherapy can use diet and nutrition adjustments as an alternative treatment

    d. Significant negative correlations exist between fast food consumption and depressive symptoms

16. Which of these statements is the most likely relationship between nutrition and depression?

    a. Cardio-protective fats (PUFA and MUFA) have no effect on depression risk

    b. Depression severity reduces with higher intake of sweet foods and fast-food/savoury snacks

    c. Inflammatory status is normal among depressed patients

    d. Trans Fatty Acid (TFA) intake is a well-known risk factor for cardiovascular diseases and depression.

17. Which of these statements best explains the relationship between depression and nutrition?

    a. Diet rich in processed meat, chocolates, sweet desserts, fried food, and refined cereals decreases vulnerability to depression

    b. Consumption of fruits, vegetables, and fish affords no protection against the onset of depressive symptoms

c. Fast food and high-fat dairy products increase vulnerability to depression

d. Higher depression severity is significantly associated with lower Mediterranean diet score (indicating a poorer diet quality).

18. Which of the following is the most appropriate recommendation on nutrition and mental health in adolescents?

a. Eating more fish could lead to reduced depressive symptoms through modification of inflammatory process

b. Improvements in mental health are not associated with improvements in diet quality

c. Reduction in diet quality bears no association with declining psychological functioning

d. Micronutrient deficiencies and malnutrition have no impact on the physical and mental development of a child

19. Which of the following has the most appropriate positive association with chronic stress?

a. Better tumour clearance

b. Cardiovascular disease

c. Improved immune functioning

d. Improved psychological functioning

20. Which of these statements best explains the role of stress as an exacerbating factor in illness?

a. Integration of a diet rich in antioxidants helps reduce the damage of oxidative stress caused by psoriasis

b. Levels of perceived stress due to IBS are significantly higher in patients treated with the mindfulness-based cognitive therapy intervention

c. Possible correlation of irritable bowel syndrome with affective spectrum disorders has not been shown

d. There is currently no evidence of oxidative stress in migraine pathophysiology

21. Which of these statements most appropriately characterizes the impact of stress on work satisfaction, immune function, and surgical outcomes?

a. Perceived patient complexity has been linked to increasing primary care physicians' work satisfaction

b. Physicians feel well-equipped to provide the socio-economic interventions patients truly need, contributing to increased stress

c. Stress reduction techniques in the elderly improve immune function with less tendency for catching flu

d. Surgical patients with higher stress levels and poor coping skills have better outcomes.

22. The concept of 'Necessary Suffering' includes:

   a. Death and separation from those we love

   b. Murder and slander

   c. Stealing and death

   d. Terrorism and separation from loved ones

23. Which of these statements best defines stress?

   a. 10% what is happening and 90% our way of looking at what is happening

   b. 50% what is happening and 50% our way of looking at what is happening

   c. 90% what is happening and 10% our way of looking at what is happening

   d. 100% what is happening and 0% our way of looking at what is happening

24. Which of these statements best explains how we create suffering for ourselves?

   a. Accepting that some pain is inevitable in life

   b. Engaging in eudaimonic thoughts

   c. Judging ourselves and others mercifully

   d. Repeating stories about our past suffering repeatedly

25. Which of these defines mindfulness?

   a. A space of awareness in which one can witness and investigate the activities of their neighbour's mind and body

   b. Being judgemental on purpose and striving with one's spouse

   c. Deep in our thoughts and unable to notice how those thoughts are driving our emotions and behaviour

   d. Developing the potential to experience each moment with serenity and clarity

26. Attitudes of mindfulness are best characterized by which of the following?

   a. Letting be, striving, and non-judging

   b. Non-judging, striving, and patience

   c. Patience, letting be, and non-judging

   d. Striving, having a beginner's mind, and acknowledging

27. Which of these statements is the most appropriate way for doctors to help patients manage their suffering?

   a. Attending closely to their own suffering

   b. Being present at domestic abuse scene to witness for themselves

   c. Ignoring their own mental state and focusing on the job

   d. Helping patients come to terms with their suffering by boasting about their own suffering

28. Which of these best characterizes some of the benefits of mindfulness-based stress reduction (MBSR)?

   a. Erodes psychological hardiness
   b. Greater energy and enthusiasm for life
   c. Increased ability to argue
   d. Loneliness among the elderly

29. Which of these is the most appropriate statement about mindfulness-based stress reduction (MBSR)?

   a. Can exacerbate loneliness among the elderly
   b. Can help people come to terms with things the way they are
   c. Can help promote 'burnout' and hedonia
   d. Has not been proven to enhance empathy amongst clinicians

30. Which of these statements best explains the effect of mindfulness-based stress reduction (MBSR) on Fibromyalgia (FM) and breast cancer patients?

   a. Immune-inflammatory pathways may in part predict the clinical efficacy of MBSR
   b. MBSR has no measurable clinical efficacy in patients with FM
   c. MBSR has no significant immune-regulatory effects in FM patients
   d. MBSR has no significant effect on emotional wellbeing, physical functioning, and overall quality of life among breast cancer patients or survivors

Answers

1. **D** Stressed people more frequently eat palatable non-nutritious food such as chips and soda (Groesz et al. 2012).

2. **C** People reporting greater stress most often report greater drive to eat (Groesz et al. 2012).

3. **C** Muscle tension, sleep disturbance, and irritability are symptoms of generalized anxiety disorder.

4. **A** Markedly diminished interest or pleasure in all, or almost all, activities most of the day, nearly every day, significant weight loss when not dieting or weight gain, or decrease or increase in appetite nearly every day and a slowing down of thought and a reduction of physical movement (observable by others, not merely subjective feelings of restlessness or being slowed down) are some symptoms of depression (Alshawwa et al. 2019).

5. **B** The PHQ-4 is a four-questionnaire answered on a four-point Likert-type scale. Its purpose is to allow for ultra-brief and accurate measurement of core symptoms/signs of depression and anxiety by combining the two-item measure consisting of core criteria for depression, as well as a two-item measure for anxiety, both of which have independently been shown to be good brief screening tools (Kroenke et al. 2009).

6. **D** The PHQ-4 is a valid ultra-brief tool for detecting both anxiety and depressive disorders. The PHQ-4 correlates well with age, gender, partnership, household income, education level, and employment status. Scores are rated as normal (0–2), mild (3–5), moderate (6–8), and severe (9–12; Kroenke et al. 2009).

7. **D** Volunteering for meaningful causes, Tai Chi, mindfulness exercises are some non-pharmacological stress management strategies (Kelly and Shull 2019, p. 238).

8. **C** Learning time management skills and relaxation therapy are useful lifestyle skills that can help in mild depression (Kelly and Shull 2019, p. 238).

9. **A** Assertiveness and problem-solving skills, improving one's sense of humour and time management techniques are healthy coping skills for emotional well-being (Kelly and Shull 2019, p. 238).

10. **A** Lifestyle medicine tackles the modifiable factors in mental health (see Tips Box 8.1).

11. **A** Evidence support hypothalamic–pituitary–adrenal axis dysregulation as an important biological link between depression and type 2 diabetes mellitus. Diabetes and depression have a bi-directional association.

TIPS BOX 8.1   Diet and Stress

- Diet and nutrition can be used as a part of a comprehensive strategy for the prevention of depressive problems.
- There are significant negative correlations between fresh fruit and depressive symptoms, but significant positive correlations between ready-to-eat food (fast food) and depression symptoms
- Chronic stress is positively associated with cardiovascular disease but negatively associated with tumour clearance and better psychological and immune functioning
- Clinicians need to attend closely to their own suffering, be present and witness their own mental state rather than striving to dispel or ignore them

Source: Adapted from Huang et al. (2019) and Kelly and Shull (2019).

Depression is associated with a flatter or blunted diurnal cortisol curve which predicts incident diabetes (Joseph and Golden 2017).

12. A Persistent major depressive disorder (MDD) and persistent generalized anxiety disorder (GAD) significantly increases the risk of incident CAD. Positive change in MDD and GAD is associated with reduced risk of incident CAD (Liu et al. 2019).

13. A SSRIs have side effects, such as serotonin syndrome, QT prolongation (for some SSRIs), bleeding, and increased risk of suicide during the early stages of treatment, among other side effects; however, there's proven efficacy of SSRIs in treating depressive symptoms in CAD. SSRIs also significantly reduce the risk of myocardial infarction in depressed patients with CAD (Fernandes et al. 2020).

14. A Orthostatic hypotension can be a problem when using TCA; however, a 2019 study suggests that there is no marked difference in CVD risks among subjects using SSRIs and non-SSRIs, for the events of MI, HF, AF, and ischaemic stroke. These findings should give confidence in prescribing non-SSRI antidepressants for patients who may not respond to SSRIs or have unacceptable side effects related to their use (Almuwaqqat et al. 2019).

15. C Diet and nutrition can be used as a part of a comprehensive strategy for the prevention of depressive problems. Moreover, patients with depression who are not suitable for drug therapy or psychotherapy can use diet and nutrition adjustments as an alternative treatment. There are significant negative correlations between fresh fruit and depressive symptoms, but significant positive correlations between ready-to-eat food (fast food) and depression symptoms (Huang et al. 2019).

16. **D** Trans Fatty Acid TFA intake is a well-known risk factor for cardiovascular disease. Depression and fatigue both have been associated with increased inflammatory activation of the immune system affecting both the periphery and the central nervous system (CNS; Lee and Giuliani 2019).

17. **D** Depression severity and current depression diagnosis are associated with unhealthy dietary intake and worse dietary quality, higher intake of sweet foods and fast-food/savoury snacks, and a lower Mediterranean diet score (MDS), respectively (Paans et al. 2019).

18. **A** Micronutrient deficiencies and malnutrition can impact the physical and mental development of a child. There is significant evidence linking diet (quality, eating pattern, and specific nutrients) and mental health among children and adolescents (Khanna et al. 2019).

19. **B** Chronic stress is positively associated with cardiovascular disease but negatively associated with tumour clearance and better psychological and immune functioning (Kelly and Shull 2019).

20. **A** Levels of perceived stress were significantly lower for the MBCT intervention compared with dialectical behavior therapy or positive psychotherapy, and diet rich in antioxidants help reduce the damage of oxidative stress caused by psoriasis. Studies show a possible correlation of irritable bowel syndrome with affective spectrum disorders (Tripathi et al. 2018; Mohamadi et al. 2019).

21. **C** Physicians feel ill-equipped to provide the socioeconomic interventions patients truly need, contributing to increased stress and perceived patient complexity has been linked to decreased primary care physicians' work satisfaction (Weiner et al. 2019).

22. **A** Illness, death, and separation from those we love are 'Necessary Suffering' (Kelly and Schull 2019, p. 244).

23. **A** Stress can be thought of as 10% what is happening and 90% our way of looking at what is happening (Kelly and Schull 2019, p. 243).

24. **D** Repeating stories about our past suffering repeatedly only causes unnecessary suffering (Kelly and Schull 2019, p. 244).

25. **D** Mindfulness is developing the potential to experience each moment, no matter how difficult or intense, with serenity and clarity. A space of awareness in which one can witness and investigate the activities of one's mind and body (Kelly and Schull 2019, p. 245).

26. **C** Patience, letting be, having a beginner's mind and non-judging are attitudes of mindfulness (Kelly and Schull 2019, p. 245).

27. **A** Doctors need to attend closely to their own suffering, be present, and witness their own mental state rather than striving to dispel or ignore them.

28. **B** Greater energy and enthusiasm for life, increased psychological hardiness, and increased ability to relax are some benefits of MBSR techniques (Alsubaie et al. 2017).

29. **B** Mindfulness can reduce loneliness among the elderly, help prevent burn-out, and enhance empathy amongst clinicians (Alsubaie et al. 2017).

30. **A** MBSR has significant effect on emotional wellbeing, physical function, and overall quality of life among breast cancer patients or survivors. MBSR has significant immune-regulatory effects in FM patients (Andrés-Rodríguez et al. 2019; Zhang et al. 2019).

References

Almuwaqqat, Z., Jokhadar, M., Norby, F.L. et al. (2019). Association of antidepressant medication type with the incidence of cardiovascular disease in the ARIC study. *Journal of the American Heart Association* 8 (11): e012503.

Alshawwa, I.A., Elkahlout, M., El-Mashharawi, H.Q., and Abu-Naser, S.S. (2019). An expert system for depression diagnosis. *International Journal of Academic Health and Medical Research (IJAHMR)* 3 (4): 20–27.

Alsubaie, M., Abbott, R., Dunn, B. et al. (2017). Mechanisms of action in mindfulness-based cognitive therapy (MBCT) and mindfulness-based stress reduction (MBSR) in people with physical and/or psychological conditions: a systematic review. *Clinical Psychology Review* 55: 74–91.

Andrés-Rodríguez, L., Borràs, X., Feliu-Soler, A. et al. (2019). Immune-inflammatory pathways and clinical changes in fibromyalgia patients treated with Mindfulness-Based Stress Reduction (MBSR): a randomized, controlled clinical trial. *Brain, Behaviour, and Immunity* 80: 109–119.

Fernandes, N., Prada, L., Rosa, M.M. et al. (2020). The impact of SSRIs on mortality and cardiovascular events in patients with coronary artery disease and depression: systematic review and meta-analysis. *Clinical Research in Cardiology* 110 (2): 1–11. https://doi.org/10.1007/s00392-020-01697-8. Epub 2020 Jul 2. PMID: 32617669.

Groesz, L.M., McCoy, S., Carl, J. et al. (2012). What is eating you? Stress and the drive to eat. *Appetite* 58 (2): 717–721.

Huang, Q., Liu, H., Suzuki, K. et al. (2019). Linking what we eat to our mood: a review of diet, dietary antioxidants, and depression. *Antioxidants* 8 (9): 376.

Joseph, J.J. and Golden, S.H. (2017). Cortisol dysregulation: the bidirectional link between stress, depression, and type 2 diabetes mellitus. *Annals of the New York Academy of Sciences* 1391 (1): 20.

Kelly, J. and Shull, J. (2019). Foundations of Lifestyle Medicine: Lifestyle Medicine Board Review Manual, 2e, 231–257. American College of Lifestyle Medicine.

Khanna, P., Chattu, V.K., and Aeri, B.T. (2019). Nutritional aspects of depression in adolescents-a systematic review. *International Journal of Preventive Medicine* 10: 42. https://doi.org/10.4103/ijpvm.IJPVM_400_18. PMID: 31057727; PMCID: PMC6484557.

Kroenke, K., Spitzer, R.L., Williams, J.B., and Löwe, B. (2009). An ultra-brief screening scale for anxiety and depression: the PHQ–4. *Psychosomatics* 50 (6): 613–621.

Lee, C.H. and Giuliani, F. (2019). The role of inflammation in depression and fatigue. *Frontiers in Immunology* 10: 1696.

Liu, H., Tian, Y., Liu, Y. et al. (2019). Relationship between major depressive disorder, generalized anxiety disorder and coronary artery disease in the US general population. *Journal of Psychosomatic Research* 119: 8–13.

Mohamadi, J., Ghazanfari, F., and Drikvand, F.M. (2019). Comparison of the effect of dialectical behaviour therapy, mindfulness based cognitive therapy and positive psychotherapy on perceived stress and quality of life in patients with irritable bowel syndrome: a pilot randomized controlled trial. *Psychiatric Quarterly* 90 (3): 565–578.

Paans, N.P., Gibson-Smith, D., Bot, M. et al. (2019). Depression and eating styles are independently associated with dietary intake. *Appetite* 134: 103–110.

Tripathi, G.M., Kalita, J., and Misra, U.K. (2018). A study of oxidative stress in migraine with special reference to prophylactic therapy. *International Journal of Neuroscience* 128 (4): 318–324.

Weiner, J.Z., McCloskey, J.K., Uratsu, C.S., and Grant, R.W. (2019). Primary care physician stress driven by social and financial needs of complex patients. *Journal of General Internal Medicine* 34 (6): 818–819.

Zhang, Q., Zhao, H., and Zheng, Y. (2019). Effectiveness of mindfulness-based stress reduction (MBSR) on symptom variables and health-related quality of life in breast cancer patients—a systematic review and meta-analysis. *Supportive Care in Cancer* 27 (3): 771–781.

CHAPTER 9

The Role of Connectedness and Positive Psychology

Introduction

The health care provider should understand how healthy lifestyle behaviours support mental health and emotional wellbeing in contemporary practice. This chapter tests the candidates' understanding of the impact of a healthy lifestyle on emotional and mental health. The questions test the concepts of positive psychology, connectedness, eudaimonia, and hedonia on wellbeing and behaviour change.

1. Which of the following options is most associated with high social media use?

    a. Low depressive symptoms
    b. Higher family and friend support
    c. Panic disorder symptoms
    d. Reduction in delinquent behaviours

Lifestyle Medicine: Essential MCQs for Certification in Lifestyle Medicine, First Edition.
Ifeoma Monye, Adaeze Ifezulike, Karen Adamson and Fraser Birrell.
© 2022 John Wiley & Sons Ltd. Published 2022 by John Wiley & Sons Ltd.

2. Which of the following options best outlines the effect high Instagram/Snapchat use has on friendship competence?

    a. Higher close friendship competence

    b. Lower close friendship competence

    c. Lower friendship support network

    d. No noticeable effect on close friendship competence

3. The effect of social media on emotional distress is best characterized by which of the following?

    a. Has the same effect on emotional distress regardless of gender

    b. Time spent on social media did not show a significant effect on emotional distress

    c. Time spent on social media has a stronger relationship with emotional distress among girls

    d. Time spent on social media has a stronger relationship with emotional distress among boys

4. Active social media users (SMUs) share life experiences like video content. Passive users (or 'lurkers') tend to observe and maintain low engagement with other users. Which of these statements best describes the effect on wellbeing on the different types of social media users?

    a. Active SMUs experience increased social support from close friends than passive SMU

    b. Active SMUs experience more social anxiety than passive SMUs

    c. Active SMUs experience poorer wellbeing than passive SMUs

    d. Active SMUs is the dominant activity on social media sites

5. Which of these best explains the association of passive social media use ('lurking'), active social media use (SMU), and depression?

    a. An active SMU is associated with lower depression

    b. Adolescents have an information-seeking and opinion-exchange approach to social media

    c. Adults have a more recreational and social approach to social media

    d. Passive social media use is associated with increased depression

6. In the 'Good genes are nice, but joy is better' 2017 study, which of these best explains the clue to healthy and happy lives?

    a. Close relationships have the same effect as money or fame on health

    b. Our relationships have an insignificant effect on our health

    c. Taking care of our physical bodies is vanity

    d. Tending to our relationships is a form of self-care

7. Which of these indicators is the best predictor of a long and happy life?
   a. Close relationships
   b. Genes
   c. Intelligence quotient (IQ)
   d. Social class

8. Which of these statements best describes the impact of mindfulness on positive emotions?
   a. Assertive coping skills are not enhanced by mindfulness
   b. College students who practice mindfulness report lower stress levels
   c. Loving-kindness meditation has no measurable effect on positive emotions
   d. Mindfulness meditation has no significant effect on positive emotions

9. Which of these pairs is/are represented in Seligman's PERMA model of Positive Psychology?
   a. Engagement and marriage
   b. Meaning and accomplishment
   c. Positive emotion and responsibility
   d. Relationship and mindfulness

10. Which of these pairs of dimensions are representative of the concept of eudaimonic wellbeing (EWB)?
    a. Autonomy and purpose in life
    b. Autonomic and sympathetic activation
    c. Personal goals and environmental factors
    d. Positivity and self-criticism

11. Eudaimonia is best characterized by which of the following statements?
    a. Cognitive-behavioural strategies are ineffective in the promotion of eudaimonia
    b. Eudaimonia is positively associated with depression in adults
    c. Eudaimonia wellbeing (EWB) protects mental health
    d. EWB may be improved by encouraging 'should' and 'must' thinking

12. Which one of these statements best describes Hedonia?
    a. Hedonia is concerned with realization of personal potential
    b. Hedonia is sometimes defined as a way of behaving
    c. Hedonia is striving for higher quality and higher standards in one's behaviour
    d. Hedonia refers to people's experience of life in positive ways

13. Which of these statements best defines hedonia?
    a. Happiness comes from inherent meaning and purpose
    b. Happiness is characterized by the presence of positive emotions and absence of negative emotions
    c. Hedonia is pursuing personal goals and maturing as a human being
    d. Hedonia is striving for higher quality and higher standards in one's behaviour and performance

14. Which of these statements best describes Eudaimonia?
    a. Eudaimonia encourages antibody synthesis gene downregulation
    b. Eudaimonia is associated with upregulation of pro-inflammatory genes
    c. Eudaimonia leads to engagement of higher cortical functioning
    d. Eudaimonia leads to overactivation of the amygdala

15. Which of these are practical habits for emotional wellbeing?
    a. Counting blessings and fault-finding
    b. Expressing dissatisfaction and speaking your mind at all times
    c. Regularly practicing acts of kindness
    d. Writing down ways people have offended you

16. Which of these activities are best used to enhance wellbeing?
    a. Dwelling on our partner's weaknesses
    b. Saying something positive to someone as opposed to something negative
    c. Undertaking an activity of self-criticism
    d. Writing a daily gratuity journal

17. Which of these statements best describes the concept of positive psychology?
    a. Increasing awareness of positive psychology plays a non-significant role in mental health nursing
    b. Positive psychology interventions are often costly and ineffective
    c. Positive psychology is the scientific study of exploring people's vices
    d. Positive psychology promotes stronger cohesion in teams in terms of valuing each other

18. Which of these best describes psychological wellbeing during a lockdown in a pandemic?
    a. Psychological symptoms (stress, anxiety, and depression) have been shown to rise in tandem with time spent in lockdown
    b. Reduced social contact and feelings of isolation have been historically linked to improved wellbeing

c. Restrictions and lifestyle changes during lockdown have been associated with better psychological wellbeing

d. Time spent in quarantine during previous disease outbreaks has been shown to have positive psychological effects

19. Ultra-processed food (UPF) is energy-dense, high in unhealthy types of fat, refined starches, free sugars and salt, and poor sources of protein, dietary fibre, and micronutrients. Which of these best characterizes the relationship between mood and UPF?

a. An increased rate of depression occurs in a linear dose-response curve with higher trans-fat intake

b. Depression is positively associated with intake of mono- and poly-unsaturated fats

c. Depression was 40% more likely to develop in adults who denied themselves fast food

d. There is a negative association between UPF consumption and the risk of depression

20. Which of these statements best describes the relationship between healthy food and wellbeing?

a. Food consumption, particularly of fruits and vegetables, is associated negatively with increased wellbeing

b. People who believe that they can make choices to change their wellbeing are less likely to endorse activities thought to enhance wellbeing

c. The consumption of fruits and vegetables in a mindful way with others represents a daily activity that people can engage in to increase their wellbeing

d. The more strongly we adopt a view that our wellbeing is under our control and can be changed, the poorer is our hedonic and eudaimonic wellbeing

21. Which of these statements best characterizes the relationship between optimism and health?

a. Higher optimism is associated with increased likelihood of healthy aging

b. Optimism and coping are predictors of reduced anxiety, distress, and depression

c. Optimism is an unmodifiable health asset

d. Optimism is a statistically insignificant predictor of depression

22. Which of these statements best explains the relationship between eating fruits and vegetables (FV) and eudaimonic wellbeing?

a. Complex nature of carbohydrates found in FV provides no effect on brain chemistry or affect

    b. Consumption of vitamin C, antioxidants, and B vitamins in FV may improve wellbeing by increasing the synthesis of neurotransmitters such as dopamine

    c. FV consumption also predicted higher negative affect and less motivation to complete tasks

    d. People who eat more FV have more intense dampening of curiosity and creativity compared with those who eat less FV

23. Which of these is a true predictor of wellbeing?

    a. Sleep quality is less strongly associated with better wellbeing than sleep quantity

    b. Trouble concentrating and shorter duration sleep are related to higher wellbeing

    c. Having good dietary habits (as indicated by fruit consumption) has no effect on wellbeing

    d. Feeling more refreshed after waking up, having less trouble concentrating, and eating more servings of fruit are indicators of daily flourishing

24. High total intake of fruits and vegetables, and some of their specific subgroups including berries, citrus, and green leafy vegetables, may best promote higher levels of which of the following?

    a. Increase incidence of psychological distress

    b. Lead to ambiguity and cancer fatalism

    c. Promote pessimism and self-efficacy

    d. Protect against depressive symptoms

25. Which of the following best describes a therapeutic lifestyle change intervention?

    a. Exercise and stress management

    b. Service to others by pointing out their faults

    c. Time in nature to ruminate over injustice by spouse

    d. Toxic relationships to learn how to be resilient

26. Hope theory is an aspect of positive psychology which centres on the processes and outcomes of goal-oriented thinking and how this thinking leads to achievement of personal goals. Which one of these options best characterizes features of Hope Theory?

    a. Higher levels of hope suggest increasing despair and subsequent apathy when contemplating goals

    b. Hope theory has a place in community settings for all people, regardless of psychopathology or physical impairment

    c. Low levels of hope drive one to a stronger inclination for goal setting and attainment

d. Low levels of hope bear no significance on one's ability to identify and achieve goals and make necessary health-related changes

27. Post-Traumatic Growth (PTG) is a positive change following a traumatic experience in which the individual is able to recognize personal strengths, achieve improvements in relationships, experience increased appreciation in life, identifying new possibilities and pursuits, and positive spiritual change. Which of these sentences most accurately explains the interaction of PTG on wellbeing?

a. Higher levels of resilience are associated with higher levels of both PTG and PTSD

b. Hope and resilience have insignificant effect on the outcome of wellbeing after traumatic experiences such as natural disasters

c. Hope is associated with higher levels of PTG and lower levels of PTSD

d. Hope predicts more severe PTSD symptoms due to disappointments and failed expectations

28. Which of these options best characterizes personal therapeutic lifestyle change intervention?

a. Counselling session with behaviour therapist

b. Pharmacotherapy with anti-depressants

c. Recreation and relaxation with family

d. Starvation and time in nature

29. Which of these statements best characterizes the concept of positive psychology?

a. The study of being fully absorbed into the present moment with a blissful immersion

b. The study of positive behavioural patterns seen in people such as courage and honesty

c. The study of critical thoughts about one's self and hope for the future

d. The study of the effects of positive emotions such as self-consciousness and introspectiveness

30. Which of these statements best defines healthy habits for emotional wellbeing?

a. Dwelling on your weaknesses and ruminating over your failures

b. Interacting with family and friends regularly face to face and over social media

c. Savouring the unpleasantness of our neighbour

d. Writing down episodes of criticism from the boss

31. Which of these statements most accurately describes the relationship between a mostly plant-based diet and emotional wellbeing?

a. Depression is negatively associated with mono- and poly-unsaturated fats

b. Fast food eaters are less likely to be dissatisfied with life and therefore have lower incidence of depression

    c. Fish oil categorically treats depression and enhances wellbeing

    d. Higher trans-fat intake is associated with happiness and reduced incidence of depression

32. Which of these statements best characterizes the benefits of a mostly plant-based diet on emotional wellbeing?

    a. Associated with increased work absences and reduced productivity due to constipation

    b. Associated with increased curiosity and creativity in young adults

    c. Leads to higher anxiety and stress scores in men

    d. Leads to excess vitamins which have been found to inhibit the feel-good hormone dopamine

33. Which of these is the most appropriate description of the relationship between physical activity and emotional wellbeing?

    a. Enhancing physical activity is an effective prevention strategy for depression

    b. Exercise has been shown to be better than psychotherapy in treating depression

    c. Routine physical activity in childhood has no effect against depression in adulthood

    d. Studies show that exercise is better than pharmacotherapy in treating depression

34. Which of these statements best explains the relationship between passive and mentally active sedentary behaviours and physical activity with depression?

    a. Passive sedentary behaviours may lessen the risk of depression in adults

    b. Substituting 30 minutes of passive sedentary behaviour with 30 minutes of mentally active sedentary behaviour has no effect on the odds of depressive symptoms

    c. Substituting passive with mentally active sedentary behaviours, light activity, or moderate-to-vigorous activity reduce depression risk in adults

    d. Substituting passive with mentally active sedentary behaviours enhances negative rumination seen in people with depression.

35. Which of these statements best explains the relationship between wellbeing and exercise?

    a. Exercise can act as a distraction from psychosocial factors such as stressful life events and may improve self-esteem

    b. Passive sedentary behaviours may lessen the risk of depression in adults by preserving brain function

c. Substituting common passive sedentary behaviours with light physical activity or moderate-to-vigorous activity may enhance depressive symptoms in adults due to tiredness

d. Substituting common passive sedentary behaviours with mentally active sedentary behaviours has negligible effect on depressive symptoms in adults

36. Which one of these best explains the association between physical activity and wellbeing of young people?

a. Physical activity appears to be an ineffective intervention for reducing depression/depressive symptoms in young people

b. Physical activity has negative mental health outcomes for children and youth through reduction in self-esteem

c. Physical activity in childhood and adolescence is associated with improved concurrent symptoms of depression, particularly when undertaken regularly and with vigour

d. Physical activity in childhood offers no protection against depression as a young adult

37. Which of these definitions is most accurate about flourishing?

a. It is a socio-psychological concept influenced by financial and business factors

b. It is a state in which a person behaves psychologically and socially awkwardly

c. It is being within an optimal range of human functioning associated with hedonia and ambivalence

d. It is defined as the combination of social, emotional, and psychological wellbeing

38. Which of these best characterizes flourishing?

a. Flourishing individuals have less satisfactory interpersonal relationships in general

b. Flourishing is composed of optimism, resilience, self-esteem, engagement, competence, meaning, and positive relationships

c. Flourishing is defined as a state in which one is unable to make a meaningful contribution to society

d. People who are flourishing are more likely to be dissatisfied with their lives and critical of their own abilities

39. Which of these statements is/are most accurate about school connectedness, nature connectedness, and emotional health?

a. Individuals who are connected to nature are more likely to be disadvantaged psychologically

    b. Nature connectedness may benefit emotional health because it provides a route through which basic psychological needs can be met

    c. Neuroticism has the strongest negative relation with adolescent emotional distress

    d. School connectedness has no measurable impact on adolescent life satisfaction

40. Which of these statements best relays the relationship between mindfulness, connection to nature, and wellbeing?

    a. Cultivating a strong bond with the natural environment may be a distraction to developing mindfulness skills

    b. Mindfulness and connection to nature counteract feelings of isolation and contribute to wellbeing

    c. Mindfulness meditation in nature can decrease the benefits of nature exposure by increasing negative mood

    d. Mindfulness meditation in nature can discourage stronger connection to nature

41. Which of these best explains the outcome from positive psychology practices such as gratitude and mindfulness practices?

    a. Improved immune function and cognitive capacity

    b. Lower self-efficacy and self-control

    c. Neuroplasticity and higher body mass index

    d. Poor medication adherence and raised inflammatory markers

42. Which of these is most accurate of people who report greater number of happy moments?

    a. Detest use of seat belts and stay married

    b. Eat fast food and drink alcohol in moderation

    c. Have anti-social behaviours and better work productivity

    d. More prone to exercise and not smoke

Answers

1. C   High social media is associated with higher depressive symptoms, panic disorder symptoms, delinquent behaviours, family conflict, as well as lower family and friend support (Vannucci and Ohannessian 2019).

2. A   High Instagram/Snapchat use predicts higher close friendship competence and friend support as compared to low social media use (Vannucci and Ohannessian 2019).

3. C   The effect of social media on emotional distress differed by gender as time spent on social media had a stronger relationship with emotional distress among girls (Thorisdottir et al. 2019).

4. A   Active SMUs create text, audio, or video content, and respond frequently to other users, which may increase social capital from acquaintances or emotional support from close friends and lead to improved wellbeing (Escobar-Viera et al. 2018).

5. D   Passive SMU is associated with increased depression, whereas active SMU is associated with lower depression. It might be that individuals with depressive symptoms use SM more passively due to depression features, such as anhedonia (Escobar-Viera et al. 2018).

6. D   Taking care of your body is important. Tending to your relationships is a form of self-care too. Close relationships, more than money or fame, are what keep people happy throughout their lives (Mineo 2017).

7. A   Ties from close relationships are better predictors of long and happy lives than social class, IQ, or even genes (Mineo 2017).

8. B   Analysis of daily emotion reported over a nine-week period showed significant gains in positive emotions regardless of meditation type (Weinstein et al. 2009; Fredrickson et al. 2017).

9. B   Seligman's PERMA model of positive psychology refers to positive emotions, engagements, relationship, meaning, and accomplishment. They provide a guide on finding and securing individual happiness (Seligman 2012; Feng et al. 2020).

10. A   Six interrelated dimensions of Eudaimonic wellbeing are autonomy, purpose in life, positive relations, self-acceptance, personal growth, and environmental mastery (Ryff 2014).

11. C   EWB may be improved by specific interventions such as acceptance and commitment therapy, mindfulness, positive psychotherapy, or other positive interventions. EWB protects mental health (Brandel et al. 2017).

12. D   Hedonia focuses on people's experience of life in positive ways while eudaimonia is concerned with realization of personal potential. Eudaimonia is sometimes defined as a way of behaving whereas hedonia is defined as a way of feeling (Huta and Ryan 2010; Pancheva et al. 2020).

13. B   Happiness is characterized by the presence of positive emotions and absence of negative emotions, and this is the hedonia perspective. All the other options characterize eudaimonia (Huta and Ryan 2010; Pancheva et al. 2020).

14. C   Eudaimonia is associated with downregulation of pro-inflammatory genes, encourages antibody synthesis gene upregulation, leads to engagement of higher cortical function, and leads to less activation of the amygdala (Kelly and Shull 2019).

15. C   Counting blessings, expressing appreciation, regularly practicing acts of kindness, and writing down how one wants to be remembered are habits for emotional wellbeing (Kelly and Shull 2019).

16. B   Examples of wellbeing-enhancing activities are consciously saying something positive to someone as opposed to something negative, writing a daily gratitude journal, or undertaking an activity of self-compassion (Macfarlane and Carson 2019).

17. D   Positive psychology is the scientific study of exploring people's strengths. These range of simple and effective positive psychology interventions when used regularly increase the individuals' wellbeing and may promote stronger cohesion and more effective teams in terms of valuing each other (Macfarlane and Carson 2019).

18. A   Psychological symptoms (stress, anxiety, and depression) have been shown to rise in tandem with time spent in lockdown (Ingram et al. 2020).

19. A   An increased rate of depression occurs in a linear dose-response curve with higher trans-fat intake (Gómez-Donoso et al. 2020).

20. C   Food consumption, particularly of fruits and vegetables, is associated positively with increased wellbeing, especially when taken in a mindful way with others. People who believe that they can make choices to change their wellbeing are more likely to endorse activities thought to enhance wellbeing and tend to have better hedonic and eudaimonic wellbeing (Holder 2019).

21. A   Higher optimism is associated with increased likelihood of healthy aging, is a modifiable health asset, and is a statistically significant predictor of depression. Optimism and coping are predictors of anxiety, distress, and depression (James et al. 2019; Fasano et al. 2020).

22. B   Consumption of vitamin C, antioxidants, and B vitamins in FV may improve wellbeing by increasing the synthesis of neurotransmitters such as dopamine. FV consumption also predicts higher positive affect and more motivation to complete tasks (Conner et al. 2015).

23. D   Feeling more refreshed after waking up, having less trouble concentrating, and eating more servings of fruit are indicators of daily flourishing. The other options are incorrect (Bartonicek et al. 2020).

24. D High total intake of fruits and vegetables, and some of their specific subgroups including berries, citrus, and green leafy vegetables protect against depressive symptoms (Głąbska et al. 2020).

25. A Service to others, exercise, stress management, time in nature, and nurturing caring relationships are therapeutic lifestyle interventions that promote wellbeing (Kelly and Shull 2019).

26. B Hope theory has a place in community settings for all people, regardless of psychopathology or physical impairment. Higher levels of hope are associated with a stronger inclination for goal setting and attainment (Duncan et al. 2020).

27. C Hope and resilience are associated with higher levels of PTG and lower levels of PTSD (Long et al. 2020).

28. C Recreation and relaxation with family are the only personal therapeutic intervention on the list. Therapeutic lifestyle changes like time in nature, service to others, nutrition, and diet can be as effective as psychotherapy and pharmacotherapy (Kelly and Shull 2019).

29. B It is the study of positive behavioural patterns seen in people such as courage and honesty. Positive emotion is the ability to view the past, present, and future in a positive manner. Engagement is being fully absorbed in the present moment with a 'blissful immersion' (Kelly and Shull 2019).

30. B Interacting with family and friends regularly face to face and over social media, writing down how one wants to be remembered, thinking of one's happiest day frequently are some healthy habits for emotional wellbeing (Kelly and Shull 2019).

31. A Depression is negatively associated with mono- and poly-unsaturated fats. Depression is higher in those who eat fast food and tranfat meals. Studies are not conclusive that fish oil treats depression (Bodnar and Wisner 2005; Kelly and Shull 2019).

32. B Plant-based meals are associated with increased eudemonic feelings and behaviour (curiosity and creativity) in young adults. It leads to improved health, quality of life, and productivity in the workplace (Bodnar and Wisner 2005; Kelly and Shull 2019).

33. A Enhancing physical activity is an effective prevention strategy for depression (Choi et al. 2019).

34. C Substituting 30 minutes of passive sedentary behaviour with 30 minutes of mentally active sedentary behaviour reduced the odds of depressive symptoms and clinician-diagnosed MDD by 5% and substituting passive with mentally active sedentary behaviours might reduce negative rumination, which, in turn, may counteract the vicious cycle of maladaptive cognitions often seen in people with depression (Hallgren et al. 2019).

35. A Substituting common passive sedentary behaviours with mentally active sedentary behaviours, or (preferably) with light physical activity or moderate-to-vigorous activity reduces depressive symptoms in adults. Psychosocial factors are also relevant; exercise can act as a distraction from stressful life events, improve self-esteem, and may reduce negative attentional biases (Hallgren et al. 2019).

36. C PA in childhood and adolescence is associated with improved concurrent symptoms of depression, particularly when undertaken regularly and with vigour (Korczak et al. 2017; Dale et al. 2019; Kelly and Shull 2019).

37. D Flourishing is defined as the combination of social, emotional, and psychological wellbeing, a socio-psychological concept influenced by social and psychological factors. It is defined as a state in which a person behaves psychologically and socially well. It is defined as being within an optimal range of human functioning associated with wellness, performance, growth, and resilience (Eraslan-Capan 2016).

38. B Flourishing is composed of positive emotions, emotional stability, vitality, optimism, resilience, self-esteem, engagement, competence, meaning, and positive relationships. People who are flourishing are more likely to be satisfied with their lives, aware of their abilities and eager to achieve, thrive, and make a meaningful contribution to society. Flourishing is defined as a state in which one functions psychologically and socially well. Flourishing individuals have more satisfactory interpersonal relationships in general (Eraslan-Capan 2016)

39. B Individuals who are connected to nature are more likely to be flourishing and functioning well psychologically. Nature connectedness benefits emotional health because it provides a route through which the basic psychological needs can be met. Neuroticism was found to have the strongest positive relation with adolescent emotional distress whereas school connectedness was the strongest indicator of adolescent life satisfaction (Kim et al. 2019; Pritchard et al. 2020).

40. B Mindfulness meditation in nature can increase the benefits of nature exposure by reducing negative mood. Cultivating a strong bond with the natural environment may be conducive to developing mindfulness. Mindfulness and nature relatedness counteract feelings of isolation and contribute to wellbeing (Nisbet et al. 2019).

41. A Greater self-efficacy, self-control, adherence, inflammatory markers, immune function, cognitive capacity, and neuroplasticity and lower body mass index are some of the findings with sustained practice of positive psychology skills such as gratitude (Lianov et al. 2019).

42. D People who experience greater number of happy moments are more prone to exercise, not smoke, use seat belts, eat well, drink alcohol in moderation, stay married, and have prosocial behaviours and better work productivity (Lianov et al. 2019).

References

Bartonicek, A., Wickham, S.R., Pat, N. et al. (2020). Sleep quality, ability to concentrate, and fruit consumption suffice to predict young adult well-being: Findings from Bayesian predictive projection, Preprint (Version 1) available at Research Square. https://doi.org/10.21203/rs.3.rs-28472/v1 (accessed 01 June 2020).

Bodnar, L.M. and Wisner, K.L. (2005). Nutrition and depression: implications for improving mental health among childbearing-aged women. *Biological Psychiatry* 58 (9): 679–685.

Brandel, M., Vescovelli, F., and Ruini, C. (2017). Beyond Ryff's scale: comprehensive measures of eudaimonic well-being in clinical populations. A systematic review. *Clinical Psychology & Psychotherapy* 24 (6): O1524–O1546.

Choi, K.W., Chen, C.Y., Stein, M.B. et al. (2019). Assessment of bidirectional relationships between physical activity and depression among adults: a 2-sample mendelian randomization study. *JAMA Psychiatry* 76 (4): 399–408.

Conner, T.S., Brookie, K.L., Richardson, A.C., and Polak, M.A. (2015). On carrots and curiosity: eating fruit and vegetables is associated with greater flourishing in daily life. *British Journal of Health Psychology* 20 (2): 413–427.

Dale, L.P., Vanderloo, L., Moore, S., and Faulkner, G. (2019). Physical activity and depression, anxiety, and self-esteem in children and youth: an umbrella systematic review. *Mental Health and Physical Activity* 16: 66–79.

Duncan, A.R., Jaini, P.A., and Hellman, C.M. (2020). Positive psychology and hope as lifestyle medicine modalities in the therapeutic encounter: a narrative review. *American Journal of Lifestyle Medicine* https://doi.org/10.1177/1559827620908255.

Eraslan-Capan, B. (2016). Social connectedness and flourishing: the mediating role of hopelessness. *Universal Journal of Educational Research* 4 (5): 933–940.

Escobar-Viera, C.G., Shensa, A., Bowman, N.D. et al. (2018). Passive and active social media use and depressive symptoms among United States adults. *Cyberpsychology, Behavior, and Social Networking* 21 (7): 437–443.

Fasano, J., Shao, T., Huang, Hh. et al. Optimism and coping: do they influence health outcomes in women with breast cancer? A systemic review and meta-analysis. *Breast Cancer Res Treat* 183, 495–501 (2020). https://doi.org/10.1007/s10549-020-05800-5

Feng, X., Lu, X., Li, Z. et al. (2020). Investigating the physiological correlates of daily well-being: a PERMA model-based study. *The Open Psychology Journal* 13 (1): 169–180.

Fredrickson, B.L., Boulton, A.J., Firestine, A.M. et al. (2017). Positive emotion correlates of meditation practice: a comparison of mindfulness meditation and loving-kindness meditation. *Mindfulness* 8 (6): 1623–1633.

Głąbska, D., Guzek, D., Groele, B., and Gutkowska, K. (2020). Fruit and vegetable intake and mental health in adults: a systematic review. *Nutrients* 12 (1): 115.

Gómez-Donoso, C., Sánchez-Villegas, A., Martínez-González, M.A. et al. (2020). Ultra-processed food consumption and the incidence of depression in a Mediterranean cohort: the SUN Project. *European Journal of Nutrition* 59 (3): 1093–1103.

Hallgren, M., Owen, N., Stubbs, B. et al. (2019). Cross-sectional and prospective relationships of passive and mentally active sedentary behaviours and physical activity with depression. *The British Journal of Psychiatry*, 2020 Aug 217 (2): 413–419. https://doi.org/10.1192/bjp.2019.60. Erratum in: Br J Psychiatry. 2020 Aug;217(2):459. PMID: 30895922.

Holder, M.D. (2019). The contribution of food consumption to well-being. *Annals of Nutrition and Metabolism* 74 (2): 44–52.

Huta, V. and Ryan, R.M. (2010). Pursuing pleasure or virtue: the differential and overlapping well-being benefits of hedonic and eudaimonic motives. *Journal of happiness studies* 11 (6): 735–762.

Ingram, J., Maciejewski, G., and Hand, C.J. (2020). Changes in diet, sleep, and physical activity are associated with differences in negative mood during COVID-19 lockdown. *Frontiers in Psychology* 11: 2328. https://doi.org/10.3389/fpsyg.2020.588604. 2020 Sep 2;11:588604. Erratum in: Front Psychol. 2020 Oct 21;11:605118. PMID: 32982903; PMCID: PMC7492645.

James, P., Kim, E.S., Kubzansky, L.D. et al. (2019). Optimism and healthy aging in women. *American Journal of Preventive Medicine* 56 (1): 116–124.

Kelly, J. and Shull, J. (2019). Foundations of Lifestyle Medicine: Lifestyle Medicine Board Review Manual, 2e, 315–322. American College of Lifestyle Medicine.

Kim, E.K., Furlong, M.J., and Dowdy, E. (2019). Adolescents' personality traits and positive psychological orientations: relations with emotional distress and life satisfaction mediated by school connectedness. *Child Indicators Research* 12 (6): 1951–1969.

Korczak, D.J., Madigan, S. and Colasanto, M., (2017). Children's physical activity and depression: a meta-analysis. *Pediatrics,* 139(4).

Lianov, L.S., Fredrickson, B.L., Barron, C. et al. (2019). Positive psychology in lifestyle medicine and health care: strategies for implementation. *American Journal of Lifestyle Medicine* 13 (5): 480–486.

Long, L.J., Bistricky, S.L., Phillips, C.A. et al. (2020). The potential unique impacts of hope and resilience on mental health and well-being in the wake of Hurricane harvey. *Journal of Traumatic Stress* 33 (6): 962–972. https://doi.org/10.1002/jts.22555. Epub 2020 Jun 29. PMID: 32598564.

Macfarlane, J. and Carson, J. (2019). Positive psychology: an overview for use in mental health nursing. *British Journal of Mental Health Nursing* 8 (1): 34–38.

Mineo, L. (2017). Good genes are nice, but joy is better. *The Harvard Gazette* https://news.harvard.edu/gazette/story/2017/04/over-nearly-80-years-harvard-study-has-been-showing-how-to-live-a-healthy-and-happy-life/ (accessed 20 Apri 2021).

Nisbet, E.K., Zelenski, J.M., and Grandpierre, Z. (2019). Mindfulness in nature enhances connectedness and mood. *Ecopsychology* 11 (2): 81–91.

Pancheva, M.G., Ryff, C.D., and Lucchini, M. (2020). An integrated look at well-being: topological clustering of combinations and correlates of hedonia and eudaimonia. *Journal of Happiness Studies*: 1–23. https://doi.org/10.1007/s10902-020-00325-6.

Pritchard, A., Richardson, M., Sheffield, D., and McEwan, K. (2020). The relationship between nature connectedness and eudaimonic well-being: a meta-analysis. *Journal of Happiness Studies* 21 (3): 1145–1167.

Ryff, C.D. (2014). Psychological well-being revisited: advances in the science and practice of eudaimonia. *Psychotherapy and Psychosomatics* 83 (1): 10–28.

Seligman, M.E. (2012). Flourish: A Visionary New Understanding of Happiness and Well-Being. Simon and Schuster. The PERMA model: Your scientific theory of happiness https://positivepsychology.com/perma-model/.

Thorisdottir, I.E., Sigurvinsdottir, R., Asgeirsdottir, B.B. et al. (2019). Active and passive social media use and symptoms of anxiety and depressed mood among Icelandic adolescents. *Cyberpsychology, Behavior, and Social Networking* 22 (8): 535–542.

Vannucci, A. and Ohannessian, C.M. (2019). Social media use subgroups differentially predict psychosocial well-being during early adolescence. *Journal of Youth and Adolescence* 48 (8): 1469–1493.

Weinstein, N., Brown, K.W., and Ryan, R.M. (2009). A multi-method examination of the effects of mindfulness on stress attribution, coping, and emotional well-being. *Journal of Research in Personality* 43 (3): 374–385.

CHAPTER 10

Fundamentals of Tobacco Cessation and Managing Risky Alcohol Use

Introduction

Smoking is a major cause of disease, leading to several chronic conditions such as heart disease, lung diseases including chronic obstructive pulmonary disease, chronic bronchitis, and several cancers. Smoking increases the risk of stroke, tuberculosis, certain eye conditions, and problems of the immune system like rheumatoid arthritis. Smoking harms nearly every organ of the body. More than six million deaths worldwide can be attributed to cigarette smoking each year. Despite its widespread acceptance, excessive alcohol use is causing increasing concern. Excessive alcohol use can also increase the risk of development or worsening of chronic diseases such as hypertension, heart disease, stroke, liver disease, and digestive problems. Alcohol has been implicated in several cancers like breast, mouth, throat, oesophagus, liver, and colon. The questions in this chapter play a major part in testing the candidate's understanding of identification of substance misuse, diagnosis, treatment, and counselling strategies to aid management of patients.

Lifestyle Medicine: Essential MCQs for Certification in Lifestyle Medicine, First Edition.
Ifeoma Monye, Adaeze Ifezulike, Karen Adamson and Fraser Birrell.
© 2022 John Wiley & Sons Ltd. Published 2022 by John Wiley & Sons Ltd.

1. Which of these is least likely to be an effective Anti-Relapse Medication (ARM) in Alcohol Use Disorder?

    a. Acamprosate

    b. Diazepam

    c. Disulfiram

    d. Naltrexone (oral)

2. Which of the following is the most accurate in regard to oral naltrexone?

    a. All users should have LFTs monitored regularly

    b. Should be prescribed for three months only

    c. Should be started at 25 mg daily

    d. Should be stopped if drinking persists two weeks after starting

3. With regard to Anti-Relapse Medication (ARM), which of the following statements is least accurate?

    a. ARM can be initiated in primary care

    b. ARM should only be started by Addiction specialists

    c. Buprenorphine may be used to reduce drinking alcohol in smokers

    d. Patients should be warned of unpleasant side effects if they drink alcohol while on Disulfiram

4. The severity of an AUD – mild, moderate, or severe – is based on the number of DSM-5 criteria met. Which of these is most accurate?

    a. Mild AUD is the presence of one to two symptoms on the DSM-5 list

    b. Mild AUD is the presence of two to three symptoms on the DSM-5 list

    c. Moderate AUD is the presence of three to four symptoms on the DSM-5 list

    d. Severe AUD is the presence of four to five symptoms on the DSM-5 list

5. Which of the following statements is the least accurate?

    a. Anti-relapse medication for AUD (ARM) are over-utilized by clinicians

    b. Both Acamprosate and oral Naltrexone (50 mg/d) are associated with reduction in return to drinking

    c. Offering treatment through primary care has the potential to reduce morbidity for many patients with AUDs

    d. Patients with AUD may not be willing to pursue or may not have access to specialized treatment

6. Which of the following statements is least accurate regarding Disulfiram use as an anti-relapse medication?

    a. Alcohol found in food, perfume, and aerosol sprays may also interact with Disulfiram

    b. Alcohol taken while on Disulfiram may cause flushing, nausea, palpitations, and, more seriously, arrhythmias, hypotension, and collapse

    c. Disulfiram should be started at least six hours after the last alcoholic drink consumed

    d. Ideally, a family member or carer, who is properly informed about the use of Disulfiram, should oversee the administration of the drug

7. Regarding the Alcohol Use Disorders Identification Test (AUDIT), which of the following is the most accurate?

    a. AUDIT has lower sensitivity and specificity than other diagnostic screening instruments such as the CAGE and MAST

    b. AUDIT can detect 91% of genuinely hazardous and harmful drinkers and excludes 87% of those who are not

    c. It was developed by World Health Organization for use in clinical settings to screen for people at risk of developing alcohol problems

    d. The instrument consists of nine items intended to cover three domains of hazardous drinking (quantity and frequency of use, dependence symptoms and other problems from alcohol use)

8. Which of the following is the best advice based on current guidelines for your patients who drink to keep their health risk at a low level?

    a. If you have one or two heavy drinking episodes a week, you do not increase your risk of death from long-term illness

    b. If you regularly drink as much as 14 drinks per week, it is best to drink these all in one day

    c. It is safest not to drink more than 24 drinks a week on a regular basis

    d. You should have two to three alcohol-free days a week

9. Which of the following statements is the most accurate?

    a. ARM can only be offered by non-addiction specialists

    b. ARM is less effective than addiction counselling for mild-to-moderate AUD

    c. At-risk drinkers are usually symptomatic

    d. Patients with severe recurrent AUD should receive chronic care management like any other chronic illness

10. Euan, a 69-year-old retired GP, admits to you that he is struggling to keep on top of his alcohol intake and continues to drink at least half a bottle of vodka most nights despite heartburn for which he has come to get Omeprazole from you. His wife has now left him due to his drinking and he is finding himself constantly pre-occupied with where he can get his next drink.

    According to the DMS 5 scoring, which of the following best describes his drinking?

    a. An at-risk drinker

    b. Mild AUD

    c. Moderate AUD

    d. Severe AUD

11. Which of the following is the most typical of 'Green tobacco sickness'?
    a. Nicotine replacement patches made from green leaves
    b. Smoking cigarettes stored in a green pack
    c. The green colouration of fingers resulting from smoking
    d. The nicotine is absorbed through the skin from the handling of wet tobacco leaves

12. Which of these are true for 'second-hand smoking'?
    a. It is the smoke that fills restaurants, offices, or other enclosed spaces when people burn tobacco products
    b. Second-hand smoke does not affect children
    c. Second-hand smoke does not cause serious cardiovascular and respiratory diseases
    d. There is a safe level of exposure to second-hand tobacco smoke

13. Which of the following risks associated with smoking tobacco is most accurate?
    a. Smoking causes about 50% of lung cancers
    b. Smoking does not cause cancer of the mouth
    c. Smoking increases your risk of developing more than 50 serious health conditions
    d. Smoking-related illnesses do not cause irreversible long-term damage to health

14. Which statement is the most accurate?
    a. Hundreds to thousands of young people start smoking cigarettes every day
    b. Most adult cigarette smokers do not want to quit smoking
    c. Smoking is the third leading cause of preventable death
    d. The majority of smokers cannot quit without using evidence-based treatment

15. Which of the following has been shown to be the most effective for tobacco cessation?
    a. Acupuncture
    b. Counselling
    c. Counselling and Medication together
    d. Medication

16. Which of the following statements regarding nicotine is the most accurate?
    a. All forms of tobacco have the potential to be addictive because they all contain nicotine
    b. As a stimulant, it has not been shown to increase attention, memory, information processing, and learning
    c. Nicotine does not meet the established criteria for a drug that produces addiction, specifically, dependence and withdrawal
    d. Nicotine is not as addictive as heroin and cocaine

17. Which of the following is unlikely to be a step in the counselling for tobacco cessation?

a. Advice to quit

b. Agree quit goals

c. Ask about tobacco use

d. Assess readiness to make a quit attempt

18. Regarding nicotine, which statement is the most accurate?

a. A typical cigarette contains approximately 2–2.5 g of tobacco

b. A typical cigarette contains on average 10 mg of nicotine

c. Nicotine from a smoked cigarette will reach the brain in as little as three seconds after inhalation

d. The elimination half-life of nicotine is four to five hours

19. Which of the following medications is least likely to increase long-term smoking abstinence rates?

a. Bupropion SR

b. Nicotine inhaler

c. Nicotine nasal spray

d. Varacyclovir

20. Sam, a 43-year-old man, whose wife recently gave birth, is keen to stop smoking because of his baby son.

He currently smokes 20 cigarettes a day. Which of the following would be the least appropriate treatment to initiate?

a. Clonidine

b. Nicotine replacement patch

c. Varenicline

d. Nicotine replacement Lozenges

21. Sam currently smokes 20 cigarettes a day. On reflection, you decide that it will be useful to combine treatments to ensure Sam does quit. Which of the following combinations would be the least appropriate to initiate:

a. Bupropion and NRT nasal spray

b. Quitline counselling and Nortriptyline

c. Quitline counselling and NRT nasal spray

d. Quitline counselling and Varenicline

22. The 5 Rs of Motivational Interviewing can encourage someone to consider a quit attempt. Which of the following least represents the Rs?

a. Relevance, reward, and repetition

b. Relevance, risk, and reward

c. Relevance, risk, and repetition

d. Relevance, root-cause, and repetition

Answers

1. B   Acamprosate, naltrexone, and disulfiram are all FDA-approved for alcohol use syndrome; the former two having recognized anti-craving properties (Carson-Chahhoud et al. 2020). In contrast, diazepam has no benefits in this setting.

2. C   Naltrexone should only be prescribed for up to six months (NICE 2018).

3. A   ARM should be started by addiction specialists in secondary care. Patients should be warned of the effects of drinking on disulfiram. Varenicline is the most effective pharmacotherapy for smoking cessation and also reduces alcohol use in smokers (Shen et al. 2018).

4. B   The levels of severity are shown along with the core questions in Tips Box 10.1.

5. A   Anti-relapse medication is if anything, underused, but the other statements are all supported by some evidence (Shen 2018).

6. C   There is no specific recommendation on waiting this long and doing so risks not breaking the cycle of addiction, whereas the other statements are justified (BNF 2020).

7. C   The 10-item AUDIT questionnaire was developed by WHO (Babor et al. 2001) and while having reasonable sensitivity and specificity, few tools, if any, achieve the stated figures.

8. D   Guidance differs between countries, but generally 14–21 units or less per week, not to binge and to have two or more alcohol-free days a week (OIV 2019).

9. D   The addition of chronic care management to a primary care appointment alone conferred no benefit in a large RCT (Saitz et al. 2013).

10. C   He has five symptoms, so classifies as moderate Alcohol Use Disorder (see Tips Box 10.1; DMS-5 Manual 2013).

11. D   Green tobacco sickness is a condition that is mainly affecting tobacco harvesters, prevalent in Asian and South American tobacco harvesters (Fotedar and Fotedar 2017).

12. A   'Second-hand smoke' or passive smoking affects everyone and causes the same issues as primary smoking, in a dose-dependent manner. There is emerging evidence that vaping also causes issues with second-hand particulates, albeit at a lesser order of magnitude than smoking itself (Avino et al. 2018).

13. C   Smoking causes ~80% of lung cancers, cancer of the mouth, a wide range of conditions, and irreversible damage, with risk even at low exposure levels (e.g. Bjartveit and Tverdal 2005).

14. A   Most adult smokers want to quit and do so without help or treatment (Smith et al. 2015). It is the single leading cause of preventable death.

TIPS BOX 10.1 | Alcohol Use Disorders (DSM-5)

The presence of at least two of the symptoms below indicates **Alcohol Use Disorder (AUD).**

The severity of the AUD is defined as:

Mild: The presence of two to three symptoms

Moderate: The presence of four to five symptoms

Severe: The presence of six or more symptoms

In the past year, have you:

- Had times when you ended up drinking more, or longer, than you intended?
- More than once wanted to cut down or stop drinking, or tried to, but couldn't?
- Spent a lot of time drinking? Or being sick or getting over other aftereffects?
- Wanted a drink so badly you couldn't think of anything else? **New to DSM–5**
- Found that drinking – or being sick from drinking – often interfered with taking care of your home or family? Or caused job troubles? Or school problems?
- Continued to drink even though it was causing trouble with your family or friends?
- Given up or cut back on activities that were important or interesting to you, or gave you pleasure, in order to drink?
- More than once gotten into situations while or after drinking that increased your chances of getting hurt (such as driving, swimming, using machinery, walking in a dangerous area, or having unsafe sex)?
- Continued to drink even though it was making you feel depressed or anxious or adding to another health problem? Or after having had a memory blackout?
- Had to drink much more than you once did to get the effect you want? Or found that your usual number of drinks had much less effect than before?
- Found that when the effects of alcohol were wearing off, you had withdrawal symptoms, such as trouble sleeping, shakiness, restlessness, nausea, sweating, a racing heart, or a seizure? Or sensed things that were not there?

(Grant et al. 2015)

However, most countries still have hundreds to thousands of young people starting to smoke (CDC 2020).

15. **C** Systematic reviews show that medication plus educational interventions like counselling are the most effective approach (e.g. Heydari et al. 2014).

16. **A** Tobacco plants all contain nicotine, belonging to the *Nicotiana* genus. Nicotine is highly addictive (NIDA 2020).

17. **B** See Tips Box 10.2. NICE Guideline [NG92] 2018. Stop Smoking Interventions and Services.

18. **B** Cigarettes contain ~10 mg nicotine and 0.7 g tobacco. It takes 10–20 seconds to reach the brain and is rapidly metabolized in the liver to cotinine with an elimination half-life of two hours.

19. **D** Most of these are recommended options (NICE 2018), but varacyclovir is an antiviral.

20. **A** Most of these are recommended options (NICE 2018), but while clonidine has modest efficacy, its use is limited by side effects, especially dry mouth and sedation.

21. **B** While counselling and drug intervention are recommended, nortriptyline is not (NICE 2018).

22. **D** The 5 Rs are Relevance, Risks, Rewards, Roadblocks, and Repetition (Catley et al. 2012).

TIPS BOX 10.2 | NICE Guideline [NG92] 2018. Stop Smoking Interventions and Services

1.3.1 Ensure the following evidence-based interventions are available for adults who smoke:

- behavioural support (individual and group)
- bupropion
- nicotine replacement therapy (NRT) – short- and long-acting
- varenicline
- very brief advice. **[2018]**

1.3.2 Consider text messaging as an adjunct to behavioural support. **[2018]**
1.3.3 Offer varenicline as an option for adults who want to stop smoking, normally only as part of a programme of behavioural support, in line with NICE's technology appraisal guidance on varenicline. **[2018]**
1.3.4 For adults, prescribe or provide varenicline, bupropion, or NRT before they stop smoking. **[2018]**
1.3.5 Agree a quit date set within the first two weeks of bupropion treatment and within the first one to two weeks of varenicline treatment. Reassess the person shortly before the prescription ends. **[2018]**
1.3.6 Agree a quit date if NRT is prescribed. Ensure that the person has NRT ready to start the day before the quit date. **[2018]**Source: Based on NICE NG92 (2018).

References

American Psychiatric Association (2013). *Diagnostic and Statistical Manual of Mental Disorders*, 5e, (DSM-5). Washington, DC: American Psychiatric Publishing.

Avino, P., Scungio, M., Stabile, L. et al. (2018). Second-hand aerosol from tobacco and electronic cigarettes: evaluation of the smoker emission rates and doses and lung cancer risk of passive smokers and vapers. Science of the Total Environment 642: 137–147. https://doi.org/10.1016/j.scitotenv.2018.06.059. Epub 2018 Jun 18. PMID: 29894873.

Babor, T.F., Higgins-Biddle, J.C., Saunders, J.B., and Monteiro, M.G. (2001). *AUDIT: The Alcohol Use Disorders Identification Test: Guidelines for Use in Primary Care*, 2e. Geneva, Switzerland: World Health Organization.

Bjartveit, K. and Tverdal, A. (2005). Health consequences of smoking 1–4 cigarettes per day. Tobacco Control 14: 315–320.

BNF (2020). https://bnf.nice.org.uk/drug/disulfiram.html (accessed 31 December 2020).

Carson-Chahhoud, K.V., Smith, B.J., Peters, M.J. et al. (2020). Two-year efficacy of varenicline tartrate and counselling for inpatient smoking cessation (STOP study): a randomized controlled clinical trial. PLoS One 15 (4): e0231095. https://doi.org/10.1371/journal.pone.0231095. PMID: 32348306; PMCID: PMC7190140.

Catley, D., Harris, K.J., Goggin, K. et al. (2012). Motivational Interviewing for encouraging quit attempts among unmotivated smokers: study protocol of a randomized, controlled, efficacy trial. BMC Public Health 12: 456. Published 2012 Jun 19. doi:https://doi.org/10.1186/1471-2458-12-456.

CDC (2020). Smoking and tobacco use. https://www.cdc.gov/tobacco/data_statistics/fact_sheets/fast_facts/index.htm (accessed 31 December 2020).

Fotedar, S. and Fotedar, V. (2017). Green tobacco sickness: a brief review. Indian Journal of Occupational and Environmental Medicine 21 (3): 101–104. https://doi.org/10.4103/ijoem.IJOEM_160_17.

Grant, B.F., Goldstein, R.B., Saha, T.D. et al. (2015). Epidemiology of DSM-5 alcohol use disorder: results from the national epidemiologic survey on alcohol and related conditions III. JAMA Psychiatry 72 (8): 757–766. https://doi.org/10.1001/jamapsychiatry.2015.0584. PMID: 26039070; PMCID: PMC5240584.

Heydari, G., Masjedi, M., Ahmady, A.E. et al. (2014). A comparative study on tobacco cessation methods: a quantitative systematic review. International Journal of Preventive Medicine 5 (6): 673–678.

NICE guideline [NG92] (2018). Stop smoking interventions and services. https://www.nice.org.uk/guidance/ng92/chapter/recommendations (accessed 31 December 2020).

NIDA (2020). Cigarettes and other tobacco products drug facts. https://www.drugabuse.gov/publications/drugfacts/cigarettes-other-tobacco-products (accessed 6 December 2020).

OIV (2019). Comparison of international alcohol drinking guidelines. http://www.oiv.int/public/medias/7169/oiv-report-alcohol-drinking-guidelines-collective-expertise.pdf (accessed 31 December 2020).

Saitz, R., Cheng, D.M., Winter, M. et al. (2013). Chronic care management for dependence on alcohol and other drugs: the AHEAD randomized trial. JAMA 310 (11): 1156–1167. https://doi.org/10.1001/jama.2013.277609.

Shen, W.W. (2018). Anticraving therapy for alcohol use disorder: a clinical review. Neuropsychopharmacology Reports 38: 105–116. https://doi.org/10.1002/npr2.12028.

Smith, A.L., Carter, S.M., Chapman, S. et al. (2015). Why do smokers try to quit without medication or counselling? A qualitative study with ex-smokers. BMJ Open 5: e007301. https://doi.org/10.1136/bmjopen-2014-007301.

CHAPTER 11

Sexual Health and HIV Lifestyle Medicine

Introduction

Sexual health is important for physical health and emotional wellbeing. The desire for intimacy is timeless, sexual feelings do not go away as you age. Lifestyle factors play a significant role in sexual performance. Sexual dysfunction may be a marker of future manifestation of non-communicable diseases such as cardiovascular or metabolic disease. Sexual health means more than being free from sexually transmitted infections or avoiding unwanted pregnancies. Modifiable risk factors include smoking, heavy alcohol consumption, sedentary lifestyle, obesity, poor sleep, and stress. Infection by the HIV virus is characterized by progressive destruction of the immune system, which results in recurrent opportunistic infections and malignancies, progressive debilitation, and death. Malnutrition is a major complication of HIV infection and is recognized as a significant prognostic factor in advanced disease. Antiretroviral therapy has improved the survival of patients with this virus. This has resulted in increased life expectancy and HIV patients are increasingly experiencing comorbidities such as cardiovascular risk factors and coronary heart disease. Some of the older medications used, such as the nucleoside reverse transcriptase inhibitors (zidovudine, stavudine, and didanosine) and older protease inhibitors (indinavir and lopinavir) may predispose patients to developing Type 2 Diabetes Mellitus and dyslipidaemia. Cardiovascular disease is now an important cause of death in HIV-infected patients.

Lifestyle Medicine: Essential MCQs for Certification in Lifestyle Medicine, First Edition.
Ifeoma Monye, Adaeze Ifezulike, Karen Adamson and Fraser Birrell.

This chapter tests the candidates on the role of lifestyle factors in prevention and treatment of sexual dysfunction and HIV.

1. Which of the following is the most predictable determinant of sexual dysfunction?

    a. Age

    b. Lifestyle

    c. Past experience

    d. Psychological health

2. Which of the following statements best represents the rate of erectile dysfunction in men with Type 2 Diabetes Mellitus?

    a. Estimated 9–10 times higher than those without diabetes

    b. Estimated two to three times higher than those without diabetes

    c. Estimated seven to eight times higher than those without diabetes

    d. Estimated four to five times higher than those without diabetes

3. A 42-year-old man presents with features of erectile dysfunction. Which of the following is most likely to be the cause of his ED?

    a. Age

    b. BMI of $28\,kg/m^2$

    c. Free testosterone level of $0.38\,nmol/l$

    d. Type 2 Diabetes Mellitus

4. In the Allen and Walter (2018) meta-analysis of health-related lifestyle factors and sexual dysfunction, which of the following best describes the findings?

    a. Caffeine intake was related to erectile dysfunction

    b. Current cigarette smoking but not past cigarette smoking had a dose-dependent association with erectile dysfunction

    c. Participation in physical activity was associated with a lower risk of female sexual dysfunction

    d. There was some evidence that a healthy diet was related to a lower risk of erectile dysfunction but not female sexual dysfunction

5. Which of the following are the most likely consequences of sexually transmitted infections?

    a. Reactive arthritis, conjunctivitis, urethritis, but not septic arthritis

    b. Reactive arthritis, conjunctivitis, urethritis, septic arthritis

    c. Reactive arthritis, conjunctivitis, gastroenteritis, septic arthritis

    d. Reactive arthritis, iritis, urethritis, septic arthritis

6. Which of the following are most likely to be musculoskeletal features of HIV?

    a. False positive Rheumatoid Factor/CCP, psoriasis but not psoriatic arthritis, arthralgia and bone pain, Reiter's Syndrome

    b. False positive Rheumatoid Factor/CCP, psoriatic arthritis, arthralgia and bone pain, but not Reiter's Syndrome

    c. HIV arthropathy, psoriatic arthritis, arthralgia and bone pain, Reiter's Syndrome

    d. HIV arthropathy, psoriatic arthritis, but not arthralgia and bone pain, Reiter's Syndrome

7. Which best describes how the COVID-19 pandemic has affected sexual behaviour in women?

    a. Higher desire and more frequent intercourse

    b. Higher-quality intercourse

    c. Less contraception

    d. More desire for pregnancy

8. In the HIV-HEART study, which of the following most accurately reports the findings?

    a. Study evaluated the prevalence of Lipodystrophy amongst HIV patients

    b. Study evaluated the five-year risk of Coronary Heart Disease amongst HIV patients

    c. Study evaluated the prevalence of hypertension amongst HIV patients

    d. Study evaluated cardiovascular risk factors (CRF) amongst HIV patient

9. In the HIV-HEART study, which of the following was the most common cardiovascular risk factor?

    a. Smoking

    b. High Triglycerides

    c. Low High-density lipoprotein

    d. High blood pressure

10. In the HIV-HEART study, Lipodystrophy was a sign for which of the following?

    a. Cardiac failure

    b. Metabolic syndrome

    c. Obesity

    d. Sleep apnoea syndrome

11. Which of the following is the most likely explanation for malnutrition in HIV infection?

    a. Mainly due to decreased caloric intake

    b. Mainly due to malabsorption of nutrients

    c. Mainly due to recurrent infections

    d. Multifactorial causes

12. Which of these statements best states the relationship between hormonal contraception and depression?

    a. Addition of progesterone to hormone therapy has been shown to induce a good mood in women

    b. Changes in oestrogen levels may trigger depressive episodes among women at risk of depression

    c. External progestin increase levels of monoamine oxidase, which degrades serotonin concentrations and thus potentially reduces depression

    d. Women with major depression have higher oestradiol levels than do control individuals

13. Which of these statements most appropriately reflects the connection between the use of antidepressants and contraception?

    a. Progestin-only products, including the levonorgestrel intrauterine system reduces the risk for the use of antidepressants and a diagnosis of depression

    b. Teenage users of progestin-only contraception have been found to be at less risk of using antidepressants than non-users of hormonal contraceptives

    c. Use of all types of hormonal contraceptives is negatively associated with a subsequent use of antidepressants and a diagnosis of depression

    d. Use of hormonal contraceptives was associated with subsequent antidepressant use and first diagnosis of depression at a psychiatric hospital among women living in Denmark

14. Which statement is the most appropriate concerning weight gain and contraception?

    a. Current evidence supports the concern that obese women are less compliant or at greater risk of contraceptive failure

    b. Hormonal contraceptive users may have a modest weight loss that is comparable to that of non-users

    c. Long-acting reversible contraceptives should be avoided in obese women due to adverse combination of efficacy, safety, and convenience

    d. Proper and safe contraception in obese women is extremely important to reduce unintended pregnancy

15. Which statement most appropriately explains the effect of choice of contraception on obese women?

    a. Combined hormonal contraception (CHC) is generally safe to use in overweight or obese women who are otherwise free of conditions that further increases their thromboembolic risk

    b. Coexistence of known risk factors of arterial vascular disease such as older age, smoking, hypertension, diabetes mellitus, and dyslipidaemia decreases the risk of thromboembolism to a sufficient extent to allow CHC use

    c. Current evidence shows that obese women are less compliant with and are at greater risk of contraceptive failure

    d. Long-acting reversible contraceptives hold the worst combination of efficacy, safety, and convenience for obese women

Answers

1. A When sexual function becomes an issue of concern for a particular individual, it is defined as sexual dysfunction. Problems with sexual function tend to increase with age. The other factors include illness, psychological health, past experience, biology, and education. Age is perhaps the most predictable determinant of sexual dysfunction. Next to age is lifestyle which can ameliorate or exacerbate the effects of ageing (Feldman et al. 1994, 2000; Egger et al. 2017).

2. B The rate of erectile dysfunction in men with Type 2 Diabetes Mellitus is estimated to be two-to-three times higher than those without diabetes (Selvin et al. 2007).

3. D Ageing is associated with an increase in abdominal fat mass, decrease in muscle mass, and decrease in activity levels and these all independently affect the testosterone level. In the Massachusetts Male Ageing Study, having a BMI > 28 kg/m2 doubled the incidence of ED at follow-up. True male hypogonadism is rare (Feldman et al. 1994, 2000).

4. C Sexual dysfunction is a common problem among men and women and is associated with relationship difficulties, lower quality of life as well as suboptimal functioning in individuals. In the 2018 study 'Health-Related Lifestyle Factors and Sexual Dysfunction: A Meta-Analysis of Population-Based Research', Allen et al. observed that cigarette smoking (past and current), alcohol intake, and physical activity had dose-dependent associations with erectile dysfunction. There was some evidence that a healthy diet was related to a lower risk of erectile dysfunction and female sexual dysfunction. Caffeine intake was unrelated to erectile dysfunction. Additionally, alcohol had a curvilinear association such that moderate intake was associated with a lower risk of erectile dysfunction (Allen and Walter 2018).

5. B All these manifestations can be triggered by STIs, with chlamydia often triggering reactive arthritis with or without conjunctivitis and urethritis. Gonococcal infection can also spread haematogenously and cause a septic arthritis (Kvien et al. 1994).

6. C There are protean manifestations of arthropathy in HIV, including all of these as well as vasculitis, atypical lupus, and Diffuse infiltrative lymphocytosis syndrome (DILS), a Sjögrens-like multi-system condition seen in HIV, which does not have the typical anti-Ro or anti-La antibodies (Adizie et al. 2016).

7. A A prospective study in Poland compared sexual activity and function on the same women before and during the pandemic, using the same tools (Yuksel and Ozgor 2020). Sexual desire and frequency of intercourse (2.4 vs 1.9, $P = 0.001$) significantly increased during the COVID-19 pandemic, whereas quality of sexual life significantly decreased. They also found decreased desire for pregnancy (19 (32.7%) versus 3 (5.1%), $p = 0.001$), decreased female contraception (24 versus 10, $p = 0.004$), and increased menstrual disorders. This shows there are current issues with sexual as well as physical and mental health.

8. D The HIV-HEART study utilized a prospective, cross-sectional multicentre design to evaluate the prevalence of cardiovascular risk factors and 10-year risk of coronary heart disease using the Framingham risk model (Reinsch et al. 2012).

9. A The most common CRFs were as follows: smoking (51.2%), high triglycerides (39.0%), low high-density lipoprotein cholesterol (27.5%), and high blood pressure (21.4%; Reinsch et al. 2012).

10. B Lipodystrophy was a sign of metabolic syndrome in the HIV-HEART study (Potthoff et al. 2010).

11. D In HIV infection, malnutrition is multifactorial. All of the causes mentioned play a role in combination to cause malnutrition (Salomon et al. 2002).

12. B The addition of progesterone to hormone therapy has been shown to induce adverse mood effects in women. External progestin, probably more than natural progesterone, increases levels of monoamine oxidase, which degrades serotonin concentrations and thus potentially produces depression and irritability. Changes in oestrogen levels may trigger depressive episodes among women at risk for depression and women with major depression generally have lower oestradiol levels than do control individuals (Skovlund et al. 2016; Rocha et al. 2017).

13. D Teenage users of progestin-only contraception have been found to be more frequent users of antidepressants than nonusers of hormonal contraceptives. Use of all types of hormonal contraceptives is positively associated with the subsequent use of antidepressants and a diagnosis of depression. Progestin-only products, including the levonorgestrel intrauterine system, also implied an increased risk for the use of antidepressants and a diagnosis of depression, supporting the finding that although the levonorgestrel intrauterine system primarily works locally, it also delivers levonorgestrel to the systemic circulation. Use of hormonal contraceptives was associated with subsequent antidepressant use and first diagnosis of depression at a psychiatric hospital among women living in Denmark (Skovlund et al. 2016; Rocha et al. 2017).

14. D Hormonal contraceptive users may have a modest weight gain that is comparable to that of non-users. Proper and safe contraception in obese women is extremely important to reduce unintended pregnancy. Current evidence does not support a concern that obese women are less compliant or at greater risk of contraceptive failure. Long-acting reversible contraceptives hold the best combination of efficacy, safety, and convenience for this group (Skovlund et al. 2016; Rocha et al. 2017; Tips Box 11.1).

TIPS BOX 11.1 | Contraception and Lifestyle

- Use of all types of hormonal contraceptives is positively associated with a subsequent use of antidepressants and a diagnosis of depression
- Women with major depression generally have lower oestradiol levels than do control individuals
- Proper and safe contraception in obese women is extremely important to reduce unintended pregnancy
- Current evidence does not support a concern that obese women are less compliant or at greater risk of contraceptive failure
- Long-acting reversible contraceptives hold the best combination of efficacy, safety, and convenience for this group

Source: Adapted from Skovlund et al. (2016) and Rocha et al. (2017).

---

15. **A**   Combined hormonal contraception is generally safe to use in overweight or obese women who are otherwise free of conditions that further increase their thromboembolic risk such as arterial vascular disease such as older age, smoking, hypertension, Diabetes Mellitus, and dyslipidaemia. Current evidence does not support a concern that obese women are less compliant or at greater risk of contraceptive failure. Long-acting reversible contraceptives hold the best combination of efficacy, safety, and convenience for obese women (Skovlund et al. 2016; Rocha et al. 2017).

References

Adizie, T., Moots, R.J., Hodkinson, B. et al. (2016). Inflammatory arthritis in HIV positive patients: a practical guide. *BMC Infectious Diseases* 16: 100. https://doi.org/10.1186/s12879-016-1389-2. PMID: 26932524; PMCID: PMC4774153.

Allen, M.S. and Walter, E.E. (2018). Health-related lifestyle factors and sexual dysfunction: a meta-analysis of population-based research. *The Journal of Sexual Medicine* 15 (4): 458–475.

Egger, G., Binns, A., Rossner, S., and Signer, M. (2017). Lifestyle Medicine: Lifestyle, the Environment and Preventive Medicine in Health and Disease, 3e, 393–398.

Feldman, H.A., Goldstein, I., Hatzichristou, D.G. et al. (1994). Impotence and its medical and psychosocial correlates: results of the Massachusetts male ageing study. *The Journal of Urology* 151 (1): 54–61. https://doi.org/10.1016/S0022-5347(17)34871-1. PMID: 8254833.

Feldman, H.A., Johannes, C.B., Derby, C.A. et al. (2000). Erectile dysfunction and coronary risk factors: prospective results from the Massachusetts male aging study. *Preventive Medicine* 30 (4): 328–338. https://doi.org/10.1006/pmed.2000.0643. PMID: 10731462.

Kvien, T., Glennas, A., Melby, K. et al. (1994). Reactive arthritis: incidence, triggering agents and clinical presentation. *Journal of Rheumatology* 21 (1): 115–122. PMID 8151565.

Potthoff, A., Brockmeyer, N.H., Gelbrich, G. et al. (2010). Lipodystrophy- a sign for metabolic syndrome in patients of the HIV- HEART study. *JDDG: Journal der Deutschen Dermatologischen Gesellschaft* 8 (2): 92–98. https://doi.org/10.1111/j.1610--0387.2009.07330.x. English, German. Epub 2009 Dec 14. PMID: 20002869.

Reinsch, N., Neuhaus, K., Esser, S. et al. (2012). Are HIV patients undertreated? Cardiovascular risk factors in HIV: results of the HIV-HEART study. *European Journal of Preventive Cardiology* 19 (2): 267–274. https://doi.org/10.1177/1741826711398431. Epub 2011 Feb 28. PMID: 21450595.

Rocha, A.L.L., Campos, R.R., Miranda, M.M. et al. (2017). Safety of hormonal contraception for obese women. *Expert Opinion on Drug Safety* 16 (12): 1387–1393.

Salomon, J., De, T.P., and Melchior, J.C. (2002). Nutrition and HIV infection. *British Journal of Nutrition* 87 (Suppl 1): S111–S119. https://doi.org/10.1079/BJN2001464. PMID: 11895147.

Selvin, E., Burnett, A.L., and Platz, E.A. (2007). Prevalence and risk factors for erectile dysfunction in the US. *The American Journal of Medicine* 120 (2): 151–157. https://doi.org/10.1016/j.amjmed.2006.06.010. PMID: 17275456.

Skovlund, C.W., Mørch, L.S., Kessing, L.V., and Lidegaard, Ø. (2016). Association of hormonal contraception with depression. *JAMA Psychiatry* 73 (11): 1154–1162.

Yuksel, B. and Ozgor, F. (2020). Effect of the COVID-19 pandemic on female sexual behavior. *International Journal of Gynaecology and Obstetrics* 150 (1): 98–102. https://doi.org/10.1002/ijgo.13193. Epub 2020 May 23. PMID: 32392400.

CHAPTER 12

Special Considerations

Women's and Men's Health, Epigenetics, Sickle Cell Disease and Diabetes

Introduction

Women's health has for a long time focused on sexual health and child-bearing issues, but increasingly, the place of healthy lifestyle behaviours in improving the growing crisis of lifestyle-related chronic diseases in women cannot be over-emphasized. Men's health incorporates a broad conceptualization of health, including predictors of health, wellbeing, health behaviours, and lifestyle choices. These remain the root cause of chronic diseases such as men's cancers, diabetes, as well as disturbances in sexual activities. As men continue to lag behind women in life expectancy, more attention is needed in this area than previously given.

Epigenetics is a new and emerging field of medicine that is set to change the way we manage patients. Increasing evidence shows that lifestyle factors as well as environmental factors may influence epigenetic mechanisms, e.g. DNA methylation, histone acetylation, and miRNA expression. Such lifestyle factors such as diet, physical activity, sleep, psychological stress, positive psychology, tobacco, alcohol, and substance use can change epigenetic patterns.

Sickle cell disease (SCD), the most common genetic haemolytic anaemia worldwide, results from the presence of a mutated Haemoglobin S (HbS). It is a glutamate-to-valine mutation of the sixth codon of the

Lifestyle Medicine: Essential MCQs for Certification in Lifestyle Medicine, First Edition.
Ifeoma Monye, Adaeze Ifezulike, Karen Adamson and Fraser Birrell.
© 2022 John Wiley & Sons Ltd. Published 2022 by John Wiley & Sons Ltd.

Beta-Haemoglobin allele; the homozygous genotype (HbSS) is associated with the most prevalent and severe form of the disease. Despite advances in care, median survival in advanced countries is still in the fifth decade, due to chronic complications. Median age of survival in developing countries is much less. Chronic pulmonary complications in SCD are major contributors to this early mortality, including pulmonary hypertension, venous thromboembolic disease, sleep disorders, asthma, and recurrent wheezing. Sleep apnoea is a common complication with many effects on sleep and daytime functioning. There is a high prevalence of obstructive sleep apnoea and it is an independent risk factor for diabetes, hypertension, myocardial infarction, and stroke.

Numerous research findings have dramatically changed our understanding of diabetes and supplied a novel approach to preventing, treating, and reversing diabetes using therapeutic lifestyle interventions.

This chapter tests candidates on the knowledge of the new focus and approach in the management of many chronic conditions, based on the overwhelming evidence and proof of concept, shown in several lifestyle medicine scientific publications and everyday practice of lifestyle medicine.

1. Which of the following weight-loss targets is most likely to significantly improve hot flushes in overweight/obese women?

    a. 2%

    b. 5%

    c. 10%

    d. 15%

2. Kim et al. (2020) compared lifestyle changes to metformin in the management of Polycystic Ovarian Syndrome (PCOS). Which of the following best describes their findings for Lifestyle Medicine compared to metformin?

    a. Improvement in BMI

    b. Improvement in insulin resistance

    c. Improvement in menstrual cycles

    d. Increase in pregnancy rates

3. Which of these statements is most likely to be accurate concerning men's health and lifestyle?

    a. Health-related self-stigma and masculine role norms are positive facilitators to men's health and wellbeing

    b. Men die an average of four to six years later than women

    c. Men experience less disability-adjusted life-years lost due to illness

    d. Men tend to overuse substances such as tobacco-related products and alcohol

4. Which of the following is the most appropriate statement about men's health?

   a. Many men's diets tend to be healthier and more nutritious

   b. Men eat fewer fruits and vegetables and, as a result, have lower fibre intake

   c. Men eat less red meat, dietary fats, sodium, and overall calories

   d. Men get more sleep, and the sleep they do get tends to be of superior quality

5. Which of the following is the truest statement about men's health?

   a. Health-related self-stigma and masculine role norms are positive facilitators to men's health and wellbeing

   b. Men are quick to seek treatment for both their physical and psychological symptoms

   c. Researchers have shown negative associations between elements of traditional masculinity and alcohol use

   d. Traditional masculinity is associated with higher symptoms of depression, greater stigma around treatment-seeking behaviour, and poorer coping strategies overall

6. Which of these statements is most likely to be accurate concerning men's health and lifestyle?

   a. Concept of preconception health is a motivating factor for healthy lifestyle adaptation with the potential to improve male fertility outcomes

   b. Hegemonic or traditional masculinity and social norms may encourage some men to take better care of their health

   c. Many clinics providing advice on postnatal care of the newborn, family planning, and couple's fertility are available to men

   d. Men define their roles as providers and protectors and, therefore, pay a lot of attention to their own health

7. Which of the following is the most correct statement about men's health?

   a. A holistically healthy father is a strong role model for ongoing healthy male child development

   b. Due to their masculine role norms, men tend to underuse substances such as alcohol

   c. Men experience less disability-adjusted life-years lost due to illness

   d. Men live an average of four to six years longer than women

8. Which of the following epigenetic markers was the first to be linked to lifestyle?

   a. Telomere shortening

   b. DNA methylation

   c. MicroRNA

   d. Histone acetylation

9. Which dietary component protects against cancer by affecting methylation?
   a. Butyrate from fibre
   b. Diallyl sulphide in garlic
   c. Genistein in soy products
   d. Sulforane in broccoli

10. Which of the following in the life course can epigenetic factors affect lifespan and quality of life?
   a. In utero
   b. Early life
   c. Middle age
   d. At any stage

11. Which of the following is the most common type of sleep apnoea in patients with SCD?
   a. Central sleep apnoea
   b. Complex sleep apnoea syndrome
   c. Obstructive sleep apnoea
   d. Treatment-emergent central sleep apnoea

12. Which of the following is most representative of the impact of trace minerals on SCD patients?
   a. Mild deficiency in serum 25-Hydroxyvitamin D is related to increased frequency of crises-related ER/hospital visits
   b. Those who almost never consume fish or milk have the same ER/hospital visits as those who consume the same regularly
   c. The deficiencies in trace minerals cause an increase in systemic oxidative stress
   d. Trace minerals have no association with the frequency of crisis-related hospitalizations

13. Which of the following reasons is the most appropriate explanation for exercise hyperventilation and reduced exercise tolerance amongst sickle cell disease patients?
   a. Decreased alveolar dead space
   b. Decreased anaerobic metabolism
   c. Hyperoxia
   d. Restrictive lung impairment

14. The high oxidative stress burden in SCD is most likely due to which of the following factors?
   a. Acute pro-inflammatory state
   b. Low autoxidation of sickle haemoglobin

    c. Low levels of cell-free haemoglobin

    d. Recurrent ischaemia-reperfusion injury

15. In Type 2 diabetes, which of the following best describes the effect of exercise?

    a. Contributes to weight loss

    b. Has no impact on cardiovascular risk factors

    c. Worsens blood glucose control in type 2 diabetes

    d. Worsens wellbeing

16. Which of the following best describes the outcome of a Stress Management Program in adolescents with diabetes?

    a. It improves adherence

    b. It improves coping styles

    c. It improves metabolic control

    d. It reduces diabetes-specific stress

17. Which of the following best describes the prevalence of Type 2 Diabetes Mellitus in those with Severe Obstructive Sleep Apnoea?

    a. 8%

    b. 18%

    c. 28%

    d. 38%

18. Which of the following best represents the relationship between HbA1c levels and 25-hydroxyvitamin D levels?

    a. Higher HbA1c levels are associated with higher 25-hydroxyvitamin D levels

    b. Lower HbA1c levels are associated with higher 25-hydroxyvitamin D levels

    c. Higher HbA1c levels are associated with lower 25-hydroxyvitamin D levels

    d. Lower HbA1c levels are associated with lower 25-hydroxyvitamin D levels

Answers

1. **C** Many Lifestyle Medicine approaches can help with vasomotor symptoms. A 10% weight loss has been shown to significantly improve hot flushes. Other approaches include eating less spicy food, and avoiding alcohol and hot drinks (NAMS 2015).

2. **B** Although metformin is known to improve insulin sensitivity in a study by Kim et al. (2020), LSM was shown to improve insulin resistance in comparison to metformin.

3. **D** Health-related self-stigma and masculine role norms are potential barriers to men's health and wellbeing. Men die an average of four to six years earlier than women, and men also experience more disability-adjusted life-years lost due to illness. Men tend to overuse substances such as tobacco-related products and alcohol (O'Brien et al. 2018; McCreary et al. 2020).

4. **B** Many men's diets tend to be less healthy and nutritious; they tend to eat more red meats, dietary fats, sodium, and overall calories. Men also eat fewer fruits and vegetables and, as a result, have lower fibre intake. Men also get less sleep, and the sleep they do get tends to be of inferior quality (O'Brien et al. 2018; McCreary et al. 2020).

5. **D** Men often delay seeking treatment for both their physical and psychological symptoms.

    Researchers have shown some positive associations between elements of traditional masculinity and alcohol use while traditional masculinity is associated with higher symptoms of depression, greater stigma around treatment-seeking behaviour, and poorer coping strategies overall. Health-related self-stigma and masculine role norms are potential barriers to men's health and wellbeing (Sinclair et al. 2019; McCreary et al. 2020; Tips Box 12.1).

TIPS BOX 12.1 | Men's Health and Lifestyle

- Many men's diets tend to be less healthy and nutritious
- They tend to eat more red meat, dietary fats, sodium, and overall calories
- Men also eat fewer fruits and vegetables and, as a result, have lower fibre intake
- Men also get less sleep, and the sleep they do get tends to be of inferior quality
- Men die an average of four to six years earlier than women

Source: Adapted from O'Brien et al. (2018) and McCreary et al. (2020).

6. A Men defined their roles as a provider and protector, with little attention being paid to their own health while hegemonic or traditional masculinity and social norms may encourage some men to put their health at risk. While there are many health clinics available to women, where advice in areas such as postnatal care of the newborn, family planning, and couple's fertility is provided, there are few, if any, equivalent health clinics available to men. Concept of preconception health serves as a motivating factor for healthy lifestyle adaptation with the potential to improve male fertility outcomes and general health and wellbeing, as well as the health of future generations (Sinclair et al. 2019; McCreary et al. 2020).

7. A A holistically healthy father, one who is engaged in the shared process of parenting, provides a strong role model for ongoing healthy male child development. Men die an average of four to six years earlier than women and experience more disability-adjusted life-years lost due to illness. Men tend to overuse substances such as tobacco-related products and alcohol (Sinclair et al. 2019; McCreary et al. 2020).

8. A All of these epigenetic markers have evidence linked to lifestyle, but telomere shortening was the first to be described and explored (evidence summarized in Shammas 2011). While DNA methylation and histone deacetylation are competing markers of premature ageing, the most promising regarding understanding the pathways and intervening are probably microRNAs.

9. C These all have effects mediated through increased histone acetylation, apart from genistein, which increases methylation (Tiffon 2018).

10. D Although there have been many hypotheses considering the effects of intrauterine programming on the development of obesity and other lifestyle-related diseases, as well as many studies focusing on one stage of life. There is overwhelming evidence that lifestyle and epigenetic factors are influential across the whole life course (Mancilla et al. 2020). This is an incredibly positive message for clinicians and patients involved in lifestyle medicine.

11. C Obstructive sleep apnoea is the commonest type of sleep apnoea across the populations, including in patients with SCD (Mayoclinic.org 2020).

12. C Moderate-to-severe deficiency in serum 25-Hydroxyvitamin D is related to increased frequency of crisis-related ER visits and hospitalizations (McCaskill et al. 2018).

13. D In SCD, there is increased alveolar dead space, increased anaerobic metabolism, and hypoxia (Pianosi et al. 1991).

14. D In SCD, there is a chronic pro-inflammatory state, higher autoxidation of sickle haemoglobin, elevated levels of cell-free haemoglobin, and a characteristic recurrent ischemia-reperfusion injury (Nur et al. 2011).

15. A Exercise has multiple benefits in Type 2 Diabetes Mellitus, in addition to contributing to weight loss, it improves blood glucose control, improves cardiovascular risk factors, and improves wellbeing (Chen et al. 2015; Lin et al. 2015).

16. **D** A stress management program in adolescents with diabetes has been shown to positively impact on diabetes-specific stress only (Boardway et al. 1993).

17. **C** The prevalence of Type 2 Diabetes Mellitus increases with OSA severity, from 6.6% in those without OSA to 28.9% in those with severe OSA (Kent et al. 2014).

18. **B** In a 12-week vitamin D supplementation study, a significant difference was seen in mean HbA1c and HbA1c change from baseline at differing 25-hydroxyvitamin D levels (Aljabri et al. 2010). Patients were more likely to achieve lower HbA1c levels at 12 weeks if they had higher 25-hydroxyvitamin D levels at 12 weeks.

References

Aljabri, K.S., Bokhari, S.A., and Khan, M.J. (2010). Glycemic changes after vitamin D supplementation in patients with type 1 diabetes mellitus and vitamin D deficiency. *Annals of Saudi Medicine* 30 (6): 454–458. https://doi.org/10.4103/0256-4947.72265.

Boardway, R.H., Delamater, A.M., Tomakowsky, J., and Gutai, J.P. (1993). Stress management training for adolescents with diabetes. *Journal of Pediatric Psychology* 18 (1): 29–45.

Chen, L., Pei, J.H., Kuang, J. et al. (2015). Effect of lifestyle intervention in patients with type 2 diabetes: a meta-analysis. *Metabolism* 64: 338–347.

Kent, B.D., Grote, L., Ryan, S. et al. (2014). Diabetes mellitus prevalence and control in sleep-disordered breathing: the European Sleep Apnea Cohort (ESADA) study. *Chest* 146 (4): 982–990.

Kim, C.H., Chon, S.J., and Lee, S.H. (2020). Effects of lifestyle modification in polycystic ovary syndrome compared to metformin only or metformin addition: a systematic review and meta-analysis. *Scientific Reports* 10: 7802.

Lin, X., Zhang, X., Guo, J. et al. (2015). Effects of exercise training on cardiorespiratory fitness and biomarkers of cardiometabolic health: a systematic review and meta-analysis of randomized controlled trials. *Journal of the American Heart Association* 4 (7): e002014. https://doi.org/10.1161/JAHA.115.002014. PMID: 26116691; PMCID: PMC4608087.

Mancilla, V.J., Peeri, N.C., Silzer, T. et al. (2020). Understanding the interplay between health disparities and epigenomics. *Frontiers in Genetics* 11: 903. https://doi.org/10.3389/fgene.2020.00903.

mayoclinic.org (2020). Sleep apnea. https://www.mayoclinic.org/diseases (accessed 20 December 2020).

McCaskill, M.L., Ogunsakin, O., Hottor, T. et al. (2018). Serum 25-hydroxyvitamin D and diet mediates vaso-occlusive related hospitalizations in sickle-cell disease patients.

Nutrients 10 (10): 1384. https://doi.org/10.3390/nu10101384. PMID: 30274253; PMCID: PMC6212983.

McCreary, D.R., Oliffe, J.L., Black, N. et al. (2020). Canadian men's health stigma, masculine role norms and lifestyle behaviours. *Health Promotion International* 35 (3): 535–543.

NAMS (2015). Nonhormonal management of menopause-associated vasomotor symptoms: 2015 position statement of the North American menopause society. *Menopause* 22 (11): 1155–1172.

Nur, E., Biemond, B.J., Otten, H.M. et al. (2011). Oxidative stress in sickle cell disease; pathophysiology and potential implications for disease management. *American Journal of Hematology* 86 (6): 484–489. https://doi.org/10.1002/ajh.22012. Epub 2011 May 4. PMID: 21544855.

O'Brien, A.P., Hurley, J., Linsley, P. et al. (2018). Men's preconception health: a primary health-care viewpoint. *American Journal of Men's Health* 12 (5): 1575–1581.

Pianosi, P., D'Souza, S.J., Esseltine, D.W. et al. (1991). Ventilation and gas exchange during exercise in sickle cell anaemia. *American Review of Respiratory Disease* 143 (2): 226–230. https://doi.org/10.1164/ajrccm/143.2.226. PMID: 1990932.

Shammas, M.A. (2011). Telomeres, lifestyle, cancer, and aging. *Current Opinion in Clinical Nutrition and Metabolic Care* 14 (1): 28–34. https://doi.org/10.1097/MCO.0b013e32834121b1.

Sinclair, K.I.A., Pritchard, D., and McElfish, P.A. (2019). An intersectional mixed methods approach to native Hawaiian and Pacific Islander men's health. *Asian American Journal of Psychology* 10 (3): 268.

Tiffon, C. (2018). The impact of nutrition and environmental epigenetics on human health and disease. *International Journal of Molecular Sciences* 19 (11): 3425. Published 2018 Nov 1. doi:https://doi.org/10.3390/ijms19113425.

Index

Lifestyle Medicine: Essential MCQs for Certification in Lifestyle Medicine, First Edition.
Ifeoma Monye, Adaeze Ifezulike, Karen Adamson and Fraser Birrell.
© 2022 John Wiley & Sons Ltd. Published 2022 by John Wiley & Sons Ltd.